Jacque C. Rigg

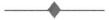

Curing
the Incurable

How to Use Your Body's
Natural Self-Healing Ability
to Overcome M.S. and Other Diseases

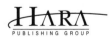

HARA
PUBLISHING GROUP

Published by
Hara Publishing
P.O. Box 19732
Seattle, WA 98109
(425) 775-7868

ISBN: 1-883697-17-4
Library of Congress Number: 98-073710

Manufactured in the United States
10 9 8 7 6 5 4 3 2

Disclaimer
The information in this book is intended for educational purposes only
and is not intended to treat any disease, nor does the author guarantee the
prevention or cure of any disease. As with any information that affects
your health, the author encourages you to discuss the information
herein with your health care provider.

Editing: Victoria McCown
Cover Design: Scott Carnz
Desktop Publishing: Scott & Shirley Fisher
Recipe Review: Cheri Tucker

Dedication

This book is dedicated to Art,
for without his
unconditional love, support and patience
I would not be walking.

My heartfelt thanks to: my new friend, Sheryn, for her very valuable input and her perseverance and dedication to getting it right; Vicki, for her courage in facing a monumental task; Cheri for her delightful sense of humor; Scott & Shirley for coping with all the corrections and additions; and Scott C. for his talent and his patience in developing the cover. I also want to thank Hazel and Louise for urging me, year after year, to get this book written and Pam and Rich for their encouragement and support after it was written. Most of all, I want to acknowledge, with love and gratitude for the tremendous joy they have brought to my life, Kathy and Teril (my daughters and my best friends), Dan, Dick, Kevin, Heather, Erin, Brian, Betsy, Meggie, and Daniel.

A Note From the Author

In spite of modern, sophisticated medicine, our society is tormented by baffling, incurable diseases such as arthritis, cancer, multiple sclerosis and a host of other maladies.

Perhaps we haven't found the right answers because we haven't been asking the right questions!

Instead of searching for cures, may I suggest that we should ask ourselves, "Why do these conditions occur in the first place?" What imbalances, shortages, and overloads occur that allow illness to overcome a normally self-repairing, self-healing organism?

When we ask the right question we get to the root of the problem and are then able to make the necessary adjustments and corrections. In other words, the solution is logical and simple. A nutrient-deprived, toxin-overloaded, out-of-balance system has no choice but to scream for help by succumbing to a diseased state. The good news: it is reversible!

Jacque Rigg

Contents

Foreward i

1 A Brief History to Get Acquainted 3

2 So Many Symptoms, So Little Time! 5

3 Enter the Knight on a White Horse 7

4 Trying to Fight an Unknown Opponent 9

5 The Day the Worms Died 13

6 A New Neurologist, a New Diagnosis 15

7 Making a Bad Tactical Decision 19

8 Macrobiotics Versus My English-Irish-French Tastebuds 23

9 More About Macrobiotics 27

10 The Diary That Saved My Sanity 29

11 Learning About Homeopathy 35

12 Mind Over Matter and Imagination Over Reality 39

13 Natural Versus Artificial 43

14 God's Great Pharmacy 47

15 On the Subject of Supplements 51

16 My Evolving Diet 55

17 Alternative Options 59

18 Reflexology and Other Safe Alternatives 65

19 A Painful Lesson 69

20 Let Food Be Your Medicine 71

21 Caffeine, Coffee, Colas and Chocolate 75

22 Healthful Substitutes 79

23 The Great Debate About Losing Weight 83

24 Your Digestive System 85

25 The Remarkable Story of Charles Benge 89

26 Combining Foods 93

27 The Fastest, Shortest Path is the Best! 97

28 A Program for Whatever Ails You 101

29 Familiar and Unfamiliar Ingredients 107

30 The Zen of Peeling, Chopping and Dicing 111

31 Two Useful Lists 113

Recipe Section: 117

Proteins 124

Neutrals 199

Starches 219

Resources: 271

Alternative Medical Associations 271

Health-Related Web Sites 277

Alternative Health Newsletters 279

Foods 280

Suggested Reading 286

Index 289

Order Form 301

Foreward

◆

In an ancient tale, a student asked the Buddha, How will I know the truth?" The Buddha replied, "Because it works."

This book is about what worked for me and why I think it will work for you. I do not have a magic potion or a quick fix for the problem of ill health. I don't know that anyone does.

Although there are hundreds of medicines that work quickly to cover up symptoms, in many cases they have simply become a part of the problem.

Western, allopathic medicine has always had a mechanical view of the human body, generally regarding us as just so many unintelligent body parts. However, I (and many others) suggest that that is NOT what we are. We contend that we are complete, complex, totally integrated, programmed, self-regulating, self-healing systems with an incredible inner intelligence. The human body is in a constant state of dynamic equilibrium, adjusting constantly to achieve a delicate balance to keep us healthy.

Conventional medicine has also maintained that certain diseases, up to now, are incurable. Therefore, if someone recovers from the incurable, many doctors are convinced that the disease has gone into remission for some mysterious, unknown reason.

However, recent studies have proven that the mind is a tremendous tool or a terrible weapon, depending on attitude. A positive, healthy outlook helps the body heal itself while pessimism can be a killer. When people are told there is no cure for their condition, many of them give up and simply wait for the disease to destroy them.

Because of my personal experience in overcoming the incurable by listening to my own inner intelligence, and because I know of others who have done the same thing, I would like to suggest that just because conventional medicine doesn't have a cure doesn't mean there isn't one.

Recognizing the awesome power of our minds, we would be wise to offer those with incurable illnesses, hope and encouragement instead of foreboding and depression.

During the stages of my recovery, I kept a diary to substantiate the fact that I did not simply go into remission. Once I discovered the proper program to reverse my steady decline, I deliberately went off my healing regimen three times, and all three times my symptoms and weakness returned.

Although I tried a great many alternative options (and, luckily, had the resources to do so), I want to assure you that the basis for my recovery from illness boiled down to three simple formulas — in a nutshell, what I ate, how I ate it, and how I utilized the power of a positive mind set.

When a genetic defect or irreversible organ or brain/nerve damage is absent, I am convinced that anyone has the potential to do exactly what I did: to overcome and *reverse* the ravages of chronic-primary-progressive multiple sclerosis. It required only the determination to get well and an acquired ability to pay attention and "listen" to my body's wisdom.

With a combination of diet, alternative healing therapies, a daily record, a "tuned-in" listening mode and the self-induced cooperation of the subconscious mind, wellness is, I believe, an attainable goal for everyone.

If I was not completely convinced that this program could work for everyone, I would never have written this book, for I would not want to give anyone false hope. On the other side of the coin, I have seen a great many people who were diagnosed as incurable give up all hope, and therefore they had absolutely no chance to heal themselves.

Please entertain the idea that I am not an exception to any rule. I did have a confirmed diagnosis (from spinal fluid) and I continued to experience the devastating effects of this disease for several years until I decided to take responsibility for my own health.

I have gone from a wheelchair-bound, totally uncoordinated, completely exhausted individual to an energetic, healthy person at age sixty-eight. I play a decent game of golf, cross-country ski, dance and walk without a hint of a limp.

So this is my story, written with the optimistic prayer that thousands of you will prove what truly miraculous beings we really are.

You'll know the truth because it works.

Chapter One

◆

A Brief History to Get Acquainted

$\mathbf{M}$y paternal grandfather was a small-town veterinarian. They called him "Doc" Eastman. He was also known as "The Stubborn Dutchman." When I was a small child, I loved to ride out to the farms with him and watch him treat sick cows and horses. He always told me that they did most of the getting well themselves. He just helped them get rid of whatever was blocking their progress toward wellness. I was proud of my grandfather for helping all those animals and was secretly pleased when someone called me stubborn. It meant I was like him.

In the years that followed, most of my time was spent in school in the winter and in the swimming pool in the summer. Swimming was great, but diving was my passion. By the time I was in high school, I was doing exhibition diving and entering some competition. At a compact five-foot two, I was blessed with good coordination and I won a number of events, including a Junior Regional AAU Championship in the Midwest. (Many years later, when I started falling down a great deal for apparently no reason, you can imagine the puzzlement!)

Married at age twenty-one, I ultimately gave birth to and raised three great children, Kathy, Dan and Teril. While living at the Champions Golf Club in Northwest Houston, I learned to play golf when I got "too old" to dive. Then, after twenty-five years of marriage, there was a typical midlife divorce, and I was suddenly on my own in a very large, scary world.

After throwing a pity party and stumbling around a considerable amount of time trying to find a way to make a living, I eventually started publishing a business newspaper in northwest Houston. The first issue came out on April 7, 1980, and during that year, I was much too busy to give any thought to several subtle, strange and persistent symptoms.

Chapter Two

◆

So Many Symptoms, So Little Time!

At first my friend Denyse noticed that I had a slight limp when we took our morning walk. I had just had quite a bout with a bad lumbar disc, so I attributed the limp to that and chose to ignore it.

Then, on several occasions after dining in a restaurant, I would stagger into chairs and walls on my way out. "Gee," I would think, "one glass of wine didn't used to affect me like this… but then, I *am* getting older."

Difficulty controlling my bladder came next, but everyone knows that as women get along in years, that often happens.

At some point my big toes started getting numb and quite often I would have tingling in my extremities. Too busy and frightened about failing in the newspaper business, I chose to ignore these clues as well.

Almost every evening I would leave my office, go home, and with the sense that something was going wrong in my body, I would fix a crunchy vegetable salad with lemon juice, sea water and cayenne, following a recipe from nutritionist Paavo

Airola's diet cookbook. Within an hour of eating my super-healthy salad, I would start experiencing the most exasperating, irritating spasms in my right leg and foot. It felt like an electric shock hit a muscle in my leg every few minutes, and my foot would draw up, toes toward my knee. This would go on an hour or so and finally fade away. Several years later I would discover that I was extremely allergic to lemon juice and that my immune system would attack me whenever I ate any food to which I was allergic. Hence, the "electric shock" symptoms.

During this period, I developed night sweats, although I was past menopause, and experienced a devastating weakness from heat. I was dropping things, falling down frequently, and most curious of all, when I lowered my chin toward my chest my thighs tingled!

Going up and down stairs was becoming extremely difficult and, even without the heat, I was exhausted all the time. Even my vision was affected occasionally, becoming blurry for several hours at a time. Can you believe, I was so engrossed in the newspaper, (and was also, by then, busy serving on the area Chamber of Commerce Board), that I still chose to ignore the fact that something was playing havoc with my body! I attributed all of this to aging!

Chapter Three

<hr>

Enter the Knight on a White Horse

Denyse, the friend who had first noticed my limp, had decided that I should meet a man that several other friends had mentioned to me. His name was Arthur Rigg, and he had just been transferred back to Houston after eight years in London. She determined this while we were sitting on her patio playing gin rummy. Houston had just experienced a sizeable hurricane and the electricity was off all over the city so I couldn't accomplish anything at my office. Denyse coerced her husband, Karl, into inviting Art out to Champions to join him and our mutual friends, the West brothers, for golf. Afterward, their wives, Denyse, and I would join the men for dinner, and Art and I would meet and put all of the matchmaking business to rest. By this time, I had decided that I was doing very well on my own, thank you, and was certainly not interested in a fifty-six-year-old bachelor, but I agreed to her plan.

He came, we met, and three months later, we married. Surprisingly, my grown children approved of this sudden turn of events, because he captured their hearts as he had mine.

In the excitement of a marvelous new romance, my health problems became quite insignificant. I can't remember much about my symptoms at that time except that I fell down once while Art and I were playing golf. Then, when we were celebrating our sudden engagement with two of his oldest friends at a restaurant, all the toasts with wine left me incapable of walking out of the place without assistance. My legs simply refused to walk, which was humiliating more than frightening.

On our honeymoon, in Hawaii, another candlelight and wine dinner resulted in my stepping off a curb and grabbing Art for support, only to knock him into the bushes on the other side of the street. I fell hard onto the pavement but, as always, broke no bones and chose to downplay the incident.

When we returned to Houston, however, all of my symptoms became more and more persistent and severe. When I walked, my right foot slapped and my right knee locked. I became almost incapable of going up and down stairs. I still had the newspaper and was trying to go to work every day, but things were coming to a head no matter how I tried to ignore them.

Chapter Four

◆

Trying to Fight an Unknown Opponent

Several weeks after Art and I returned from Hawaii, my editor, Sam, whose wife was a physician, noticed my progressively limping gait and suggested that his wife take a look, "just to be safe." I agreed, as I was exasperated with the symptoms and the fatigue.

After a cursory examination, Sam's wife tactfully suggested that I immediately see a neurologist. It seems that when she drew a pencil up the sole of my foot, from the heel to the toes, it reacted in an abnormal fashion. My toes curled up toward my knee instead of going to a point.

Upon my insistence on knowing why I should take such a step, she admitted that she felt there was a good chance that I had a brain tumor. Good grief! That certainly ruined the rest of my day.

It didn't take long before they had me in the hospital, undergoing a week's worth of tests. Most of them seemed like Chinese water torture....they went on and on and on and they aggravated my nerves, muscles and temperament.

Through it all, Art was like a mother hen, hovering, supporting, encouraging, and worrying.

Within a week after the tests concluded, the results and the diagnosis were reported. The neurologist had no earthly idea what was wrong. A brain tumor had been ruled out, thank goodness, but I was left with a terrible emptiness and frustration about doing battle with an insidious opponent that wouldn't reveal itself and yet continued to progress relentlessly, day by day.

For a few weeks, I wore an extremely uncomfortable neck brace because the tests had revealed a bad disc in my neck that the doctor felt might be causing a few of my symptoms. It wasn't.

As I traveled with Art throughout the Orient (his position required trips to the Far East, from Australia to Japan) and then returned to catch up with the newspaper business, I became even more weak and unable to walk more than a few yards at a time. I also became quite irritable every time we had to walk more than a few feet, because it felt as though someone had tied some very large lead weights to my feet.

While staying at a charming inn in Kyoto, Japan, I was so devastated by the heat of the traditional bath that I had to crawl out of the tub and back to my room. On a trip to Washington, D.C., the only way I could view the museums and galleries was for Art to push me in a wheelchair. How I hated that!

I was terribly tired from the time I got up in the morning until bedtime. Pushing myself only made things worse and, for the first time in my life, I was beginning to feel that I couldn't control anything that was happening to me.

I started reading books on health and looking for answers in every direction. I tried acupuncture. It would slightly relieve some of my symptoms for an hour or so, and then they would come roaring back.

The Chinese acupuncturist sent me to a dentist first because he had decided that I had TMJ, a problem with the jaw joint, and he wanted me fitted with a mouthpiece to wear at night. He also suggested that I might want to have my amalgam dental fillings removed. Most of my fillings had been replaced by crowns and were not exposed, so the dentist and I both felt that removal was a bit much. I settled for the mouthpiece. The acupuncturist worked with me for several months, and he also tested me for allergies. He and I were both confounded by the number of things I reacted to negatively. I, who had never appeared to be allergic to anything, reacted to what seemed like three-fourths of the world's substances. After telling me he could no longer perform acupuncture (evidently we had reached a limit of some kind), he announced in his broken, difficult-to-understand English that he had determined that I had M.S.

"Oh, no. That can't be," I said. I had undergone a battery of tests and they had ruled out M.S. He was unimpressed and assured me I definitely did have M.S.

I chose not to believe him, because a whole army of doctors and technicians belonging to our modern medical brigade had decided that I did not have M.S.! Another valuable lesson learned.. much later.

In the meantime, I had found a chiropractor that worked on me in a very gentle, nudging fashion and a massage therapist with wonderful hands. They were both knowledgeable about acupressure points and again, I felt better and could walk a bit better after their treatments, but it never lasted more than an hour or two.

Chapter Five

---◆---

The Day the Worms Died

Next came the discipline of the raw food diet. A lady who espoused eating only raw foods and drinking wheat grass juice came to Houston. I obtained a personal consultation. All that I had to do to get well, she said, was stop eating dead, cooked foods which had lost their enzymes, and eat nothing but organic, raw produce.

Not only that, but I needed to grow my own sunflower sprouts and wheat grass, using organic soil.

I spent the next few weeks buying plastic trash cans, drilling them full of holes so my earthworms could breathe, ordering earthworms from an ad in *Field & Stream*, filling the cans with garden soil, earthworms and table scraps, and setting up a shelf garden at our atrium window.

The first sprouting of sunflower seeds and wheat grass was an exciting event! Poor Art. Newly married, after having been single for so long, he had decided, I am sure, that he had wed a lunatic. He was still trying to support and encourage me, but some of my new, "spacy" friends involved in the raw food movement gave him many serious moments of doubt. Later, we decided that becoming overzealous and eating only raw foods for a considerable period of time, is too restrictive for a well-balanced diet.

I was, however, nibbling on sprouts and carrots, juicing my wheat grass, losing weight, and convinced that my body was becoming healthier every minute.

Each day I would carry our table scraps to the organic-soil trash cans, turn them in to the soil, thank the little earth worms for processing my garbage and go inside to water my sprouts.

All this time however, I was in denial and ignoring the fact that I was feeling better but my legs were getting weaker and none of my symptoms had disappeared.

Then, one day, while tending to my compost at the back door, I was horrified to discover that Houston's unbearable heat had done in my earthworms. Every last one of them was dead. No worms, no rich, organic soil. No rich, organic soil, no vitamin-packed greens. No vitamin-packed greens, no cure for whatever in the world was wrong with me.

I was devastated. There didn't seem to be anything I could do to arrest this terrible, crippling, disease with no name. I cried most of the night in Art's arms.

Chapter Six

◆

A New Neurologist, a New Diagnosis

It had been a year since my first series of tests and I was getting a great deal worse quite rapidly.

One day Art came home from work and, in his most diplomatic manner, suggested that I see another neurologist. He knew how I felt about those blasted tests but was determined that we find out, if at all possible, what was happening to me. A friend of his had highly recommended a doctor associated with the Baylor College of Medicine, who practiced at Houston's Methodist Hospital. After several days of his persistence (he can be as tenacious as a bulldog when he has made up his mind), I gave in and agreed to make an appointment with the new neurologist.

During that office visit I discovered that I couldn't balance on one foot or raise up on my toes without tipping over, that a reflex hammer whacked below my knee cap produced a reaction so violent I almost lost my new neurologist, and that he, the bruised one, was determined to put me back in the hospital for more tests.

Too exhausted to argue with Art *and* the doctor, I "turned myself in" to Methodist Hospital.

Several new tests were added to the familiar ones. They had just installed a new MRI unit, which was, at that time, the latest technology. They strapped me into a coffin-like tunnel with a constant, noisy voice and insisted that I stay there without moving (even my head was strapped down) for three straight hours. I meditated and did self-hypnosis and imagined beautiful beach scenes and golf courses for about two hours. But by then, I had endured quite enough. For the last hour, Art held my hand and talked to me while I tried very hard not to scream. Much to his relief, I made it. (I understand they have become more compassionate since then and have added earphones with music and other amenities to the MRI experience.)

My hospital stay this time became a contest of wills between me and the dietitian. She was fearful that my raw food diet was not sufficient and I was just as convinced that her sugar, white flour and canned vegetable regimen would eventually kill me. We finally compromised after several visits. She sent me large chef salads and whatever else I asked for after I revealed my stash of nuts and seeds that I was using to supplement my tray. I ate what I wanted and she gracefully stayed in the kitchen. I realize now that we were *both* locked into a belief system that was not necessarily valid. If I have learned anything of value through all of this, it is that each individual and each disease is uniquely different. You absolutely cannot generalize when it comes to what is best or what works for each individual. I cannot emphasize this enough!

The last test was a spinal tap. The pain from the subsequent headache was right up there with having babies, but it caught the culprit. A firm diagnosis: multiple sclerosis.

At last, a name was given to the enemy! My relief was tempered, however, by the fact that my roommate was diagnosed at about the same time. Hers was Lou Gehrig's disease, and my emotions nose dived as she and her family questioned the doctors about how long she might live. How I wish I had known then what I know now! I would have tried very hard to convince her not to believe them when they insisted it was incurable and fatal. I watched her accept their diagnosis and give up on living.

In my opinion, a medical diagnosis of incurable and/or fatal, even though it is based on past experience, is unreliable. The fact is, the doctor doesn't have a cure. **That does not mean that there isn't one! It just means he doesn't know what it is.**

Chapter Seven

——◆——

Making a Bad Tactical Decision

My doctor had "good" news. The problem, he said, with M.S. was that your immune system attacks the myelin sheath surrounding the nerves, which creates scar tissue, which short-circuits the message to the muscles. (They have recently discovered that the nerves are actually severed.)

He and a few other doctors were experimenting with the use of cytoxin (a chemotherapy cancer treatment) which is a very powerful immune system depressant. With this treatment, he advised, my immune system would quit attacking me, and chances were I would stop getting progressively worse.

Pleased with the prospect of having a weapon against my now-exposed enemy, I quickly agreed to return to the hospital after a few days and undergo treatment. It was to be a ten-day program with the cytoxin dripping into my veins continuously for that period.

I was warned that it might make me nauseous and that all my hair would probably fall out, but it seemed a small price to pay for a halt to the progression of this disease.

My two daughters, Kathy and Teril, came to Houston to, among other things, help me pick out a wig so that I would be prepared when I lost my hair. That escapade was a welcome relief from all the seriousness, for we laughed until we cried as we all tried on most of the wigs in the store. I ended up with a salt and pepper one, close to matching my own hair, after they convinced me it was perfect. Then it was time to go back to the hospital.

Looking back, I realized that for the previous four or five months, I had been cleaning out my system with the raw foods, wheat grass juice, enemas and colonics to the point that my body was *so* clean it went into shock as soon as the poison started invading it. Nausea and then unbelievable heartburn were continuous and only got worse each day.

By accident, I discovered that if I ate heavy, fatty foods it relieved my distress somewhat. So I, the adamant raw foods advocate, jumped on the bread and butter bandwagon and quickly determined that gravy and ice cream had become my new best friends.

After ten days they sent me home. But I had promised that I would return in six months for a checkup so they could evaluate how their experiment had worked.

What I didn't realize was that at the same time they were giving me the cytoxin, they were including something that kept me from being *really* sick! Shortly after arriving home, whatever "that" was had lost its effectiveness, and for the next two days I not only thought I was going to die, I really, really wanted to.

Sure enough, in a few weeks all my hair fell out. However, I was beginning to feel halfway decent, and my symptoms had lessened somewhat, so Art suggested that we take a relaxing trip back to Hawaii. The purpose, of course, was to forget all the bad stuff and enjoy those beautiful golf courses.

The neurologist had given me a statement of disability which meant I could get a handicap sticker for the car. Since it was also accepted at most golf courses, I was allowed to drive a cart up close to tee boxes and greens. That meant I could play golf with almost no walking. Without that indulgence I would not have been able to play at all. As it was, my coordination was so lousy I was quite a bad golfer, but that didn't matter. Playing great golf is not a high priority when compared to walking.

Denyse and Karl joined us in Hawaii, and our first golf outing was really delightful. Everything seemed to be going well until we got back to our hotel room. I had been wearing my new wig and within the hour my scalp started itching like crazy. The itching was so bad, I thought I might go completely berserk! Horrible red bumps covered my entire bald head and I could NOT keep from scratching them. It turned out that some little, local varmints called "No-See-Ums" had assumed I was ready to bio-degrade and had only tried to do their job. They had not bothered my healthy, cytoxin-less friends and husband one bit, nor anyone else I questioned the next day.

Later, I would realize that this episode was only a slight inconvenience compared to what would follow as a result of the chemotherapy.

Chapter Eight

◆

Macrobiotics Versus My English-Irish-French Tastebuds

While I was still in Methodist Hospital, another friend came to visit and left me with a book on macrobiotics. She had had some health problems, she said, and it really seemed to help. At the time, I was not open to anything other than the chemotherapy my scientific wizards had recommended and I had become totally disillusioned with the raw food discipline. I was depressed, discouraged, and feeling rotten physically and mentally.

However, I am by nature an optimist and a do-it-yourselfer, so upon our return from Hawaii, when my legs were still acting like rubber bands, I read the macrobiotic book.

Most of the information made logical sense so I decided to try some of the suggestions they made about diet for a week or two. Gung ho I went, and of course, if Art wanted to eat, he went, however reluctantly, with me.

So, there we were, doing macrobiotics. There was a Macrobiotic Center in Houston serving meals and giving counsel and I delighted in having lunch there, meeting people who had become much more healthy and had even divested themselves of several diseases by eating in this fashion. I was feeling a little better myself, so I bought several more books on the subject and had a consultation with one of their counselors, who was visiting from Boston.

He was very enthusiastic and knowledgeable and he offered me hope that I, too, could benefit from a macrobiotic diet. The only problem I had with his advice was that he suggested that I eat lots of burdock root (a very strong-tasting vegetable), hijiki (a very strong-tasting seaweed) and the stoutest miso they make (which is a soybean product). I had never tasted any of these things; in fact, I had never even heard of them. But I don't doubt that if I could have swallowed any or all of them, they might have been of some benefit. I tried very hard to cook and consume all of these strange food items, and to Art's credit, he did *not* gag and spit them back out on his plate. But I couldn't stand them and neither could he.

I decided, much later, that I should have been eased into the macrobiotic diet with all its foreign foodstuffs, instead of being given all the strongest tasting ones all at once. Nevertheless, I stuck with macrobiotics for quite some time because I didn't seem to have anywhere else to go.

The counselor had also introduced me to a treatment called "moxibustion." It entailed lighting a cigarlike stick and holding it close to some acupuncture points on my legs and back until I couldn't stand the heat anymore. This was a tortuous procedure, but Art and I gave it a two-week trial. It really wasn't worth the pain.

A trip to Disney World and Epcot Center was another low point in my year not because I didn't enjoy the sights but because I spent most of the time in a wheelchair with Art pushing me. Again, I hated the loss of independence, but I simply couldn't walk more than a few yards at a time. I resolved during that trip to do whatever it took to get well.

When we got back to Houston, it was time to make my six-month visit back to the neurologist.

Whatever attitude I have developed toward wellness and the medical profession was pretty much set in motion on that visit. First, I was reminded that the chemotherapy treatment was to be a once-a-year proposition. Then I was subjected to another spinal tap just to see how well the cytoxin had worked. While I was on the table with the needle in my spine, I told the doctor that I was on a diet that seemed to be helping. He gave me some excellent advice. "To be scientific," he pontificated, "you should keep a diary so that you can tell whether or not it really helps, then go off your diet to see if you become worse again."

He wasn't really interested in my diet any more than I was interested in going back to him every year for more cytoxin. He was simply intent on proving to me that diet wouldn't help. That was the end of our relationship.

I had already decided that there had to be a better way to try to get well than to knock out my immune system and poison every cell in my body. The whole experience was a great lesson in using my common sense and trusting my own judgement.

Chapter Nine

◆

More About Macrobiotics

I flew to Massachusetts that spring to the Macrobiotic Kushi Institute in the Berkshire Hills to see if I could learn how to cook these strange food items well enough to make them palatable. Michio and Aveline Kushi are the founders and two of the instructors at the institute.

I must say, it was a delightful experience. Their hospitality was heartwarming, the food quite appealing, and I left there, after a week, feeling better than I had in a long time. Aveline Kushi is a charming, intelligent, and dedicated tiny person. Petite as I am, I felt like I was towering over her. One evening, during a lively group discussion, I mentioned that it was very difficult for me to eat properly while traveling overseas with my husband. She told me in no uncertain terms that if I wanted to get well, I would have to get my priorities in order. First you get well, then you travel. The truth sometimes isn't what you want to hear.

I came home enthused about macrobiotics (by the way, the word means "great life") and determined to follow Aveline's advice. For the next several weeks we ate brown rice and beans and organic vegetables and a tiny amount of sea vegetables, but for some reason the miso really disagreed with me. I couldn't stand the taste of it anyway, so I gave up trying to get it down.

In the meantime, I had developed some strange new symptoms. Even my personality became affected. The inability to concentrate, poor memory, a feeling of "spaciness," sudden irritability over little things, mood swings, depression, headaches, indigestion and bloating all afflicted me at one time or another. My big toenail started turning black and anything I was exposed to containing mold made every symptom twice as bad. Red patches appeared around my hairline and on my chin. They itched constantly.

A friend who had known me for some time noticed the personality change. I had been fairly easygoing and slow to become irritated and now any tiny thing would set me off. (Thank goodness I had married a very patient man!) She brought me a book entitled *The Yeast Syndrome* and suggested that I read it, pronto. I did. It didn't take a great brain to realize that when I was given the cytoxin to suppress my immune system, a full-blown case of candida albicans yeast infection had taken over. I would fight it, along with the M.S., for the next nine years. I wanted to return to the neurologist and remind him that when he took The Hippocratic Oath, he had agreed to "Above all, do no harm!" but I didn't.

So now, many macrobiotic foods such as miso were on my "don't eat list" and my taste buds could still hardly tolerate some of the others. Also, the macrobiotic list of acceptable foods had been developed by a Japanese man who had determined that you should eat local produce as much as possible. However, in the same breath, he shunned such things as grapefruit, which I loved and which grew abundantly in south Texas.

There seemed to be but one possible solution for my dilemma and that was to find *my own* path back to health.

Chapter Ten

♦

The Diary That Saved My Sanity

To begin with, I decided that since my immune system attacked me whenever I ate something to which I was allergic, I was going to have to eliminate all those things from my diet.

How I regretted not making a list of all the foods the Chinese acupuncturist had named that seemed to be allergens for me! He had used a great many vials full of who knows what, which I held while he tested me with some kind of little electrical machine. To tell the truth, I didn't really trust his findings or his machine. (I have since become much more open-minded.) In the meantime, he had moved to Arizona and I couldn't reach him. As I slowly discovered which foods to avoid, however, I remembered that he had pinpointed each and every one much earlier.

There didn't seem to be much left on this earth that my body liked, so I bought some books about allergies to find out what could be done.

One suggestion, which I tried, was to fast for three days to rid the body of all suspected foods and then eat only one food each day. I was given several ways to determine whether or not a particular food was wrong for me. If my pulse rate quickened after eating something, that food was to go on the allergic list. If not, it was all right to eat. Since my pulse rate quickened after almost everything I ate, I would have been starving in no time. But I discovered a built in warning system that had been with me all along that allowed me to choose the worst of the culprits. My foot, which had drawn up in spastic fashion for all those years for apparently no reason, did its dance the minute I ate a real allergen such as lemon juice or soy milk.

One of the suggestions on ways to discover food allergies had been to take a niacin capsule before eating a particular food. If I reacted with a "niacin flush," I was allergic to that food item. The problem with that was that I was allergic to something in the niacin capsule, so every time I took one I experienced the flush. I became beet red, hot as blazes and I itched all over. We figured that out in no time.

In the end, after keeping my diary for a long time, I became aware that my body tingled after eating a troublemaker or I might swell up a little or have some indigestion. Once in awhile my eyes became blurry, but that usually seemed to happen outdoors, when I was exposed to a pesticide or other toxin. One of the most obvious symptoms that helped me identify the most unacceptable foods was that I had even more trouble walking within the next twenty-four hours after eating them.

Identifying all the allergens was a tedious endeavor and it took several months before my body calmed down and I discovered, for certain, which foods were causing me the most trouble. If I had not kept a diary to note symptoms, how I felt, how I walked, and what I had eaten, I would now be writing this from a wheelchair if I could write at all.

Finally, I ascertained that anything containing saturated fat was causing me no end of trouble. That included all meat (everything that ever walked or flew) and all dairy products. The meat was not so hard to give up, but the cheese! I loved cheese! For several years I kept the diary and three times after refraining from cheese and other goodies for a few months I would give another try at being scientific, as my neurologist had suggested. It was uncanny. If I went off my diet for two or three days in a row, my limp became dramatically worse. After a while my health became much more important to me than proving anything scientifically.

One thing I had learned from my raw food diet and macrobiotics was that organic, whole foods made my system purr, and processed, chemical-laden foods did not agree with me at all. It stands to reason that I am not alone in this. All the thousands of artificially manufactured food-stuffs on the market today have surely contributed greatly to the increase in cancers of all kinds, the prevalence of autoimmune disorders, and who knows what else!

Not only have we polluted our food (and our environment) with pesticides and hundreds of other poisons, we have then refined and processed the life out of it and added thousands of nonfood additives before putting it on the grocery shelves. It is not surprising that so many of us are getting sick! We have ingested so many chemicals and been deprived of so many nutrients that the surprise, to me, is that we aren't all dead! Only the most marvelous and miraculous of organisms could have coped with our outrageous destruction of the food supply and kept on functioning.

So, I started eating only whole, unprocessed food. Organic, if possible. That meant no refined flour or sugar, no canned drinks, diet or otherwise, no packaged precooked meals, no canned fruits or vegetables, no fat-free, skimmed anything. In other words, if man had messed with it I forsake it. If it was natural, produced by Mother Nature, I ate it.

Foods were not the only culprits. During this process, I tried to eliminate everything I possibly could that was causing my immune system to get upset. I drank purified water and avoided pesticides and all other chemicals as much as possible. I also kept away from crowds. Every virus I contacted set me back considerably, and I continued to have three or four viral infections every year for a number of years. If my average, healthy neighbor was laid up for one week with the prevalent bug, it would knock me out for two or three. My immune system was so screwed up I considered wearing a mask when I socialized.

Let me repeat once more that what causes me trouble is not, necessarily, what causes you trouble. (If you have multiple sclerosis, however, there is abundant evidence to show that saturated fat should be avoided.) I believe it is absolutely essential that each person chooses his/her own unique path to wellness. It takes commitment, determination, a conscious tuning in to your body, and a *record* of food intake, other exposures and symptoms to know what is helpful to you and what is harmful. (Being stubborn doesn't hurt either.) Don't think for a minute you can remember it all. You can't.

I am not the least unique in being able to tune in to my body. Anyone can do it. All you have to do is pay attention! Noticing what's going on and then writing down what you notice both become easier the more you try. When we take our health for granted and pay little attention to how food affects us (unless we are beset with a bad case of indigestion), we aren't aware of all the subtle sensations that are messages from our very cells. Your body has a built-in intelligence that will astound you. Some might call it intuition. It's a physical gut reaction, sometimes near the navel area and sometimes nearer the heart, or a feeling of lightness perhaps, for yes and a heaviness for no.

When you are testing yourself for food allergies, don't expect a complex answer from your body. Before you eat a certain food, as you eat it and afterwards, concentrate on your stomach area and silently ask, "Is this food O.K. or not O.K.?" It shouldn't take you long to start feeling a definite negative or positive signal.

Other images may come to mind as you meditate on the state of your being. Relax, breathe deeply and notice any and all quiet signals. Be sure to write them all down to assess later.

A note of caution: There is a big difference between "O.K." and an absolute craving for something! One of the things I read in an allergist's book was to write down a list of foods that

I felt I could not live without. That list, he said, probably represented my worst allergies.

There are other ways to ascertain some of your allergies, such as blood tests. Two I have heard of are the cytotoxic or the IgE/RAST test. I don't believe they can identify all of them, however. Talk to your doctor for advice.

Some allergists recommend the rotary diversified diet in which you don't repeat any given food for a given period of time. That might work a little later, but in the beginning someone who's immune system is attacking them needs to identify and avoid all allergic substances for a considerable time.

I eventually trusted myself and my O.K./ not O.K. method most of all while observing my symptoms and making notes in my diary, and it definitely worked for me. However, I would think it worked a great deal more slowly than being tested to find many of the troublemakers.

Note:

Just before this book was ready to print, I read about a revolutionary treatment used to cure allergic reactions. It is called NAET (Nambudripad Allergy Elimination Technique). A book describing NAET, which also contains the names of practitioners in the U.S. and Canada, is called:

Winning The War Against Asthma & Allergies
by Dr. Ellen Cutler, D.C.
Delmar Publishers, 1998
To order, call 1-800-842-3636

There is also a web site with a searchable directory of practitioners by geographic area:
http//www.naet.com

Chapter Eleven

◆

Learning About Homeopathy

About the time I discovered that I had a systemic (which means throughout the body) yeast infection, Art was ready to retire and we had planned to move to the hill country northwest of Austin, Texas.

My friend, who had noticed my nasty temperament and had given me the book on the subject of yeast infections, also gave me the name of a young man in Austin to turn to for help. His name was Jack Tips, a homeopath and a nutritionist.

I contacted Jack shortly after we moved, and he assisted me in many ways to overcome my afflictions. He is an intelligent, compassionate human being with an open mind. If I read about something I thought would help, he would discuss it with me and, perhaps, help me try it.

For instance, I read of a doctor in Arizona who was using a certain snake venom in minute doses to help M.S. patients. This particular venom would send a message to the nervous system to protect itself. Jack found a homeopathic remedy containing this particular venom and we tried it. It seemed to help.

But, mainly, Jack spent about two years building up my entire system, one organ at a time. We both agreed that a strong immune system was a whole lot better than a suppressed one, so we spent over a year working on that. The building-up was done with Systemic Formulas, which are a combination of vitamins, herbs and glandulars. Homeopathic remedies are a very, very diluted amount of a substance which would give me the same symptoms I was experiencing so that my body's defense mechanism would kick in.

I owe Jack a great deal. I would certainly not have improved as rapidly and steadily without him. But, again, only I could tell for certain if what he was offering was working. He helped me keep the candida under control with a liquid named Tai-ra-chi, but it wasn't until several years later that I read another book that would bring about some miraculous changes in that respect.

In the meantime, however, I was very, very slowly getting better. For several months I would notice no difference at all and then gradually I would become aware that I was able to do something better than I had before. Putting on my shoes had been a problem because I didn't have the strength in my legs to pull my feet up toward my hands. I simply had to go down to the floor where my feet were. I also had great difficulty putting on a pair of pants because I couldn't balance on one foot while raising the other one, ever-so-slightly, into a pant leg. After a few years on my new diet, however, I began to accomplish these kinds of things more and more normally.

I want to impress on you that self-healing requires patience. You probably didn't get sick overnight and you aren't going to reverse things immediately either. Our society is so dedicated to a pill or some other medicine that seems to be a quick cure. But all we are doing in most cases is covering up the message our body is trying to send us that things are going awry.

Also, you have to *believe* that you can make a big difference in your health. I have a friend who was diagnosed with M.S. at about the same time I was. Even though I saw her a number of times in the beginning of our affliction and told her what I was doing, she somehow didn't believe anything would help her. She never changed her diet or tried to eliminate her food allergies. I guess she was totally convinced by the doctors who told her M.S. was incurable. She probably also thought that I was rather crazy. She has been in a wheelchair, constantly, for a number of years and the quality of her life has diminished greatly. We all make our choices and take responsibility for our health, one way or another.

A great many other people have contacted me over the years when they hear how well I have done. It doesn't take long in our conversations for me to know whether the person is willing to make the effort to get well. Once I hear "Oh, I could never give up hamburgers!" (or whatever), I know they will accept ill health. That is, of course, their choice.

However, it breaks my heart to know, after my experience with cheese, that once you give up those favorite foods and start regaining your health, you can't remember what the big deal was about not being able to eat them. I have eaten a wholesome diet for so long that I can honestly say my food tastes a great deal better than the things I used to eat. Once your taste buds become accustomed to something as alive and utterly delicious as a fresh, organic strawberry, you wouldn't bury it under a blob of sugary whipping cream for the world.

Chapter Twelve

———◆———

Mind Over Matter and Imagination Over Reality

During all this time I was using subliminal tapes (how was I supposed to know they "didn't work"?) and imagining my body healing itself. I would instruct all my nerves to reroute, if necessary, in order to get the messages to my muscles. I figured that I was the captain of this particular ship and that if anyone could give it orders I could. My entire being was intent on getting well, and I welcomed any and all methods that might be of help.

Massages certainly felt good and I always imagined, as I was being worked on, that old toxins and stored, harmful emotions were being released, allowing new, healthy nutrients and healing thoughts to flow into the stagnant zones.

The research on laughter being a great medicine was just my cup of tea. Art has a delightful sense of humor and loves to make me laugh. I watch comedies instead of violence or tragedies, and my children and six grandchildren have been a great source of joy. It is not only great fun to laugh, it is good for you!

When we built our new house in which to retire, the builder and Art tactfully tried to convince me that an elevator was, eventually, going to be an absolute necessity. They meant well, but I refused to even consider it. To do so would have entertained the possibility that I would not get well. I compromised by letting them put a wheelchair ramp in the garage up to the kitchen. It has come in handy when someone has to bring something heavy into the house on a dolly. I haven't needed it, nor did I expect to.

What I have been talking about here is attitude. I firmly believe that your subconscious pays great attention to everything you think and everything you say. (If you don't believe me, take up golf!) When you are determined, convinced and totally optimistic about your body's ability to heal itself, I'm certain your chances improve considerably.

Know that beyond a doubt your cells would just love to get well. They only need your complete cooperation and that involves a healthful diet, adequate nutrient intake, the careful avoidance of toxic chemicals and allergens, and a positive attitude — the latter, perhaps, being the most important of all. I recently bought a book entitled *The Healing Power Of Mind*, by Tulku Thondup, a Tibetan Buddhist monk. It is a powerful and convincing argument that our spiritual selves are capable of incredible miracles. My suggestion to you is that, until you have left absolutely no stone unturned, don't accept our modern medicine's attitude about incurable illness.

One method I tried, which I now believe to be extremely important, was self-hypnosis. Earlier in my life I had been phobic about flying in airplanes and had undergone hypnosis to try to overcome the fear. My experiences while "under" made a *strong* impression on me. Our subconscious mind is unbelievably powerful! Since I had been totally cured of my fear of flying, I felt confident that my subconscious could also help me get well. So I made a self-hypnotic tape, putting myself in the completely relaxed state, then instructed my body (immune system, nerves and all) to accelerate the healing process. I played that tape (with earphones) to myself almost every night before I went to sleep for several months. There is absolutely no doubt in my mind that listening to that tape again and again was a powerful tool toward wellness.

Chapter Thirteen

◆

Natural Versus Artificial

Seven years had passed from the time I was given chemotherapy to the day I told a whole-foods, gourmet cooking teacher from New York, Annemarie Colbin, that my body had cured itself of M.S. with diet, herbs, vitamins, and mind-set. In that time studying alternative healing methods and substances had become my new passion.

Don't get me wrong, the M.S. is still lurking in there somewhere. But over the years I have become so healthy it doesn't stand a chance. I am in tune enough with my body that the minute I get a message that something isn't quite right, I right it. I can still bring back symptoms if I go off my diet through carelessness, but it takes a lot longer.

The only thing I haven't conquered is a devilish problem with the heat. I can't function outside in really hot weather. However, many of my friends near my age have the same problem.

There are so many options to good health and so many natural substances available for healing regimens that it amazes me that anyone will accept the artificial, expensive, side-effect-causing drugs promoted by the pharmaceutical companies and most doctors. The doctors have been trained to write prescriptions to mask symptoms rather than use nontoxic, natural therapies to promote true health. The drug companies spend billions to promote their products.

A good example is the barrage of ads and commercials for across-the-counter drugs. Acid reflux seems to be big right now. "When heartburn has you by the throat... take such-and-such for fast relief!" Could it be that taking better care of your stomach and altering your eating habits slightly might work better in the long run? I fear that far too many people are opting for fast relief for the moment only to be plagued by much more serious problems later on.

The same companies are using messages about prescription drugs with the suggestion that you "Ask your doctor if such-and-such a drug might not be good for you." Talk about drug pushers!

Greed and profit have undermined our health-care system to such an extent that anyone with an inexpensive, natural product or system to promote health is ostracized, hounded, defamed and/or crucified to prevent them from getting their agenda to the public.

Since a natural product cannot be patented and since drug companies spend millions getting their product patented so they can make many more billions in profit, they are not the least bit interested in promoting anything that works, has no side effects, and doesn't cost much. Not only that, the pressure they have applied on the FDA to keep these natural products off the market has been enormous and, in my estimation, criminal. They scream "quackery" continually to obscure the fact that some things have been working for generations to help people get well.

A herb called stevia, used as a natural sweetener in South America for hundreds of years with no side effects is, in some instances, a great replacement for refined sugar and those artificial sweeteners that are suspect but profitable. It is safe for diabetics, but our FDA refuses to allow it to be used by manufacturers as a sweetener in teas or foods, although artificial sweeteners can be used indiscriminately. Stevia was, for a very long time, outlawed in this country by the FDA. They finally have allowed it to be sold separately, as a supplement, so that *you* can use it to sweeten food. (You can find it in the supplement section of your health food store.) It seems expensive, but a very little bit goes a long, long way. I have used it in several of my recipes.

As far as I am concerned, our FDA does its utmost to usurp our freedom of choice when it comes to natural remedies. The original intent, when our government formed the Food and Drug Administration, was to protect us from dangerous drugs that hadn't been tested and to keep con artists from preying on naive, sick citizens. The FDA has so greatly expanded its role and been so increasingly influenced by the American Medical Association and the giant pharmaceuticals, that it doesn't seem to be the least bit interested in serving me or you. Any natural, God-given remedy that has been used with success by our ancestors should be available to us to use, at our own risk.

If you look at the records you will find that the drugs approved by the FDA have not only more side effects, but have caused the deaths of a great many "protected" citizens. The number of deaths caused by prescription drugs in this country is astounding. Thousands of citizens have drug-induced memory loss, Parkinson' symptoms, ulcers and a myriad of other adverse reactions. Thousands of car wrecks and hip fractures are due to legal drugs that sedate or cause dizziness in patients. If the father of medicine, Hippocrates, who said "Let food be your medicine" knew what was going on, I feel certain he would demand that our modern physicians take his name off their oath.

Most diseases seem to depend on a crippled, inefficient or confused immune system. The latter, as I described earlier, caused my multiple sclerosis. A suppressed, crippled or inefficient one allows horrible conditions such as cancer to take over.

Let me ask you a question. If you became mentally confused about something, do you think it would make more sense to:

A.   Locate the information you need to end your confusion? or

B.   Ask someone to hit you in the vicinity of your brain with a baseball bat?

Your brain was causing the problem. It was confused, right? Wouldn't bashing it with a bat make as much sense as "bashing" a confused immune system with poison? How about a crippled or inefficient immune system? If it allows such diseases as cancer to gain a stronghold, how about bashing it with chemicals and radiation? I can't help but wonder who first decided that poisoning people was the proper way to make them healthy.

I'm afraid that too many diehards in the medical establishment have invested far too much time, money and reputation in their answer to cancer to back off and admit it isn't working; but the truth is, their statistics are appalling. If, during all those years of applying poison to the problem, they had, instead, researched how to help the body strengthen its innate ability to fight back, how much better off do you think we might be?

The good news is that a number of doctors and researchers are using a new treatment strategy called "biotherapy" against cancer. It involves nutrients, phytochemicals, botanical medicines, immune enhancing factors, enzymes and hormones as well as some conventional therapies. Common sense takes a giant step for mankind!

As I am finishing this book, the news about future cancer treatment is good. It seems that some medical researchers decided they might be on the wrong track and have gone in a different direction. How I wish that some of them would investigate the incredible power of organic food!

Chapter Fourteen

◆

God's Great Pharmacy

I can't begin to cover all the natural herbs, essential oils, and other alternative therapies available to you in this book. I can, however, describe some of the basics that I have used with great success. One of the best books about herbs that I have found is *The How To Herb Book* by Velma J. Keith and Monteen Gordon. I have made a list of my favorites. Here they are.

Ginger – This herb is almost a pharmacy all by itself. People have been using ginger for about 5,000 years! It relieves nausea and vomiting, vertigo, dizziness, migraine headaches and it slows the heart rate but increases the force of the heart's contractions. It contains an enzyme which digests protein and is also antibacterial. It is a powerful antioxidant and, like aspirin, inhibits blood clotting. A great cold medicine, ginger is a good antihistamine, encourages the release of mucus, promotes sweating and increases circulation. It is antiviral, antifungal, anti-inflammatory and anti-diabetes among other attributes!

Buy the whole herb at the grocery store. Cook with it by grating or juicing, or make tea with it (two slices added to a cup of boiling water and simmered for fifteen minutes). Or you can make a ginger compress, a macrobiotic remedy. There is a small, inexpensive grater made especially for ginger.

It is also sold in powder form in the grocery store or in capsules at health food stores. Most practitioners recommend one gram a day in capsule form to benefit from its many curative powers.

Forget ginger ale. It is not a good way to take ginger.

Garlic — Raw garlic leaves an awful breath odor, so I take odor-free Kyolic Formula 102 two to three times a day, when necessary. Garlic is also an ancient remedy. Many call it nature's antibiotic, as it is effective against bacteria, viruses and fungus. It has successfully been used against parasites, infections, high blood pressure, tumors, warts and a host of other ailments. It is a blood cleanser, a liver detoxifier and is even active against staphylococcus, and E.coli bacteria.

Cayenne/Capsicum – This is the same hot pepper spice you use in cooking, but is available in capsule form and can absolutely work miracles. It improves the whole circulatory system and regulates the flow of blood which influences the heart. If Art or I were to have a heart attack or start to go into shock, capsicum capsules would be my first thought. It is a marvelous stimulant, normalizes blood pressure, builds up the immune system and has been used for a great variety of ailments. One warning, however: if you suffer from arthritis, it may be an irritant.

Aloe Vera – This cactus-like plant is so easy to grow, every house should have a plant or two. It is marvelous for burns, insect bites, rashes, acne, poison ivy or oak, and any other skin conditions. The juice can be taken internally for ulcers, diverticulosis, stomach aches, heartburn, colitis and a myriad of other discomforts. Exceptionally healing, aloe is found now in a great many cosmetic formulas. Unfortunately, the producer can sometimes dilute the juice with so much water as to render it ineffective. Even if it says on the bottle "100% aloe vera," the product can still be greatly diluted. So check carefully to make sure you have a pure, undiluted product.

Chlorophyll - So close in its molecular structure to the human red blood cell, hemoglobin, it is called "the blood of plant life." When I was on the raw food diet, I drank wheat grass juice. Later, I took spirulina. Then, when there was some question about its purity, I changed to Green Magma, which is freeze-dried barley grass juice. I have finally settled on alternating between Sun Chlorella, which is a green single-cell algae, (purifying, energizing, easy to swallow little tiny tablets) and Fiber Greens, which is a combination of fiber, friendly bacteria, soy, beets, broccoli, celery, carrots and parsley, an immune enhancing herb called cat's claw, and the dehydrated juices from wheat grass, barley grass, alfalfa, spirulina and blue-green algae. Chlorophyll counteracts toxins, accelerates healing, and is, I believe, one of the absolute essentials for anyone trying to find their way back to health.

Echinacea - A very popular natural antibiotic, this herb enhances the immune system and is an effective blood purifier. Used in combination with goldenseal, astragalus, yarrow, and/or cayenne it is a powerful infection fighting formula. For people with hypoglycemia, it is combined with myrrh instead of goldenseal. When my children or grandchildren start to feel under the weather, they immediately start taking echinacea. Great stuff.

Papaya – Not just an exotic fruit but a great digestive aid. Art and I have been using it for years instead of indigestion and heartburn remedies from the drugstore. It relieves gas and upset stomach and even helps when I have eaten hard-to-digest foods that cause me to have an allergic reaction. My favorite is Super Papaya Enzyme Plus. I chew three or four tablets after heavy meals as if they were breath mints. I haven't had indigestion in ages. Here, again, as with all natural remedies, it doesn't cover up symptoms as artificial drugs do, but actually helps take care of potential problems. It's a good idea for the first few weeks of a get-well program to chew a few tablets several times between meals as well as after every meal. Good digestion, as you will see later on, is an absolute *must* in eliminating disease, and the extra enzymes might help rid your body of any undigested "litter" hanging around.

Vinegar (Raw, Unfiltered, Organic Apple Cider Vinegar) – This vinegar is loaded with vitamins and minerals and rich in potassium. While it adds acid to the stomach to aid digestion, it is actually an alkaline-producing food. It has also been used as a mild antibiotic for generations.

What I Do When Colds Or Flu Sneak In — Because antibiotics are NOT effective against the viruses that cause colds and flu, and yet physicians have consistently prescribed them "in case a bacterial infection sets in," I never contact a doctor immediately when I feel a cold or the flu coming on. I have my own arsenal now, and it sometimes works quite effectively.

Sambucol is an elderberry extract formula patented by a doctor in Israel. It has been tested and proven in laboratory and clinical studies to be effective against airborne viruses. It comes in a liquid extract and a lozenge. At the first sign of symptoms I immediately start taking both.

Echinacea with astragalus or goldenseal is my next line of defense, along with extra vitamin C, zinc, garlic, extra chlorophyll, and more than the usual ginger.

I drink lots of liquids, including citrus juices and ginger tea, and I rest for two or three days.

A recent germicidal extract made from grapefruit seeds called Citricidal has been added to my medicine cabinet. The liquid form is useful in washing fruits and vegetables and the capsule form is easy to take and powerful. The overuse of antibiotics has created many drug-resistant strains of bacteria and I feel safer with my regimen than with antibiotics.

Actually, I have gone quite a long time now without succumbing to a viral infection, and I am convinced that, just as the No-See-Ums didn't attack my healthy friends in Hawaii, bacteria and viruses cannot get a foothold in a healthy body.

Important warning: If you are using natural remedies and you don't get much better within three days, see your M.D. or an alternative practitioner because a secondary bacterial infection is a possibility and conventional medicine's arsenal includes new, broad spectrum and more powerful antibiotics that can be used as a last resort.

Chapter Fifteen

◆

On the Subject of Supplements

I have mixed emotions about the subject of supplements. It is distressing to me to see the medical community, which has just recently discovered the subject of nutrition, trying to divide food into its separate parts, just as they have done with the human body. They keep promoting individual vitamins and antioxidants as if those components were not just a simple part of a complex whole, the foods you find them in. Our bodies were designed to eat the carrot, not swallow a vitamin A tablet. One of the dangers in all of this, I believe, is that our scientists have yet to recognize all of the intricate ingredients in the food Mother Nature produces. Phytochemicals are one of the latest discoveries. These are biologically active compounds in fruits and vegetables with incredible disease prevention and healing properties. The big "secret" is, that you get most all of the vitamins, minerals, phytochemicals and whatever else you need from a well-rounded diet of whole, organic foods. There is an actual, measurable **energy** in food that is not present in a vitamin capsule.

Many studies in medical journals correlate dramatic reductions in chronic degenerative and autoimmune disease as well as cancer and heart disease in those populations whose diets are high in fruits and vegetables.

Trying to eat a deplorable diet and make up for it with artificially manufactured nutrients is really foolhardy.

Having said all of that, I still think there are times when supplements may have a valid role to play in our health.

It is hard to eat enough food at times to ingest all the nutrients our bodies need to *overcome* disease. I started taking a natural vitamin-mineral supplement with plenty of the vitamin B complex to make sure that my cells had all the nutrients I could give them to repair themselves. I also believe that taking a green superfood (which is a whole food concentrate, not a segregated micronutrient) such as Fiber Greens, Green Magma, KyoGreen, or Sun Chlorella is an excellent way to supply nutritious compounds to a body trying to mend itself.

I do take a calcium citrate supplement just before bedtime to help protect my bones (and to help me sleep). At times, I will take a natural vitamin E and selenium together. I have also taken vitamin C off and on when it was lacking in my diet. I know when I'm not eating well enough (usually when traveling) and need to supplement my diet.

Hans Nieper, M.D., a specialist on M.S. forbids dairy products in the diet. He also advocates taking calcium EAP, which is part calcium and part phosphatidyl ethanolamine, a chemical found in the protective covering around nerve cells. EAP carries calcium to the nerve cell membrane where it assists the electricity involved in nerve transmissions. I take calcium EAP in tablets, although I have read that the intravenous form is far more effective. The FDA bans this form of delivery in the U.S. by enforcing a rule that an injectable form of a nutrient is equivalent to an unapproved drug. How like them!

Finally, each morning, I take a probiotic (beneficial intestinal microorganisms) as described in Chapter 28.

I used to grind up flax seed and sprinkle it on grains because so many alternative practitioners recommended it. However, I discovered that flax oil (along with organ meat and egg yolk) contains a substance called arachidonic acid. Too much of this acid can create various health problems, so I no longer use flax or recommend it.

In the beginning of my program I took evening primrose oil because several authorities considered a lack of essential fatty acids to be one of problems of people with multiple sclerosis. I switched, later, to borage oil capsules which are less expensive and contain the same nutrient.

Because I have found the proper foods to supply me with the nutrients I need, I no longer take supplements. EPA (or eicosapentaenoic acid) is found in salmon and tuna, which I eat regularly, and GLA (or gamma linolenic acid) is available in oatmeal. I not only cook oatmeal for breakfast often, but snack on oatmeal cookies when I need a comfort food (my own home-made cookies, sweetened with fruit and fruit juice).

Chapter Sixteen

◆

My Evolving Diet

It seems that a new book comes out every week or so espousing a new theory on health, diet and nutrition. Most of them are written by doctors or scientists with impressive credentials and each author is convinced, I am sure, that they have THE answer for everyone. The problem is, there is so much disagreement, especially in the diet field, and each expert is supporting a relatively narrow view of a complex subject. Also, many of the authors seem to have blinders on when it comes to anything that doesn't support their personal theory.

I am wary of anyone who tries to convince us that we ALL would do better if we followed their diet. We are all so uniquely and wonderfully different, it is hard to fit us into a universal mold or healing program.

Think about it. Our ancestors came from a variety of different areas of the world and they ate everything from whale blubber to papayas. They left us with an incredible diversity in our genetic structure creating different colors of hair, skin and eyes. Not only do we have an assortment of body shapes, our blood types vary, each one of us has fingerprints like no one else, and a DNA test can quite accurately determine our individual identities. *What **your** body recognizes as a perfect diet might prove to be a nightmare to **mine**.*

When I decided to strike out on my own and trust my own judgement, I was eating a great many whole grains (due to the macrobiotic influence). I did try, for a very short period of time to become a total vegetarian, thinking that might be the healthiest form of diet. However, my body did not agree with me. When I stopped eating fish, I had much less energy, I was hungry every few hours and my blood sugar level was like a roller coaster. I also tried to eat just fruit in the morning. That didn't work well either. Same problems.

I eventually discovered that when I ate protein early in the day I didn't have as much trouble with the blood sugar low in the afternoon that had plagued me for some time.

A real revelation came some time later when I was trying to lose a few pounds. Since my diet was already void of saturated fat and sugary treats, I surmised that to lose weight I would have to cut back on starches. That meant cutting way back on breads, grains, pasta and potatoes. For several weeks, I ate mostly protein (fish, tofu and other soy products) and the non-starchy vegetables, including lots of salads. It was actually a shock to discover that I felt much better, had more energy and had *no* blood sugar problems whatsoever. I also lost several pounds. My cravings for sweets and starches eventually disappeared completely and I have been eating that way ever since and feeling great. Since all carbohydrates turn into "sugar" before the body can use them, I had been flooding my system with lots and lots of blood sugar by ingesting all those starchy carbohydrates and, therefore, keeping my insulin levels high and then craving more sugar.

I didn't completely understand why this new way of eating totally agreed with me, but I certainly knew that it did. Then I read a book by Barry Sears, Ph.D. called *The Zone*. I have to admit that my initial reaction to his premise (which is that grains, other than oatmeal, are not an ideal food for us) was quite negative. After all, I had overcome and reversed a terrible disease with a diet containing a considerable amount of grain. Something kept nagging me about the book, however, so I reread it a few months later. It was then that I realized that my diet had evolved over a period of years and was presently almost exactly the same as the one he suggested. By paying attention to the reactions of my body to food, I had stumbled into "the zone" on my own. The only disagreement I have now with Dr. Sears is that for the initial few months of eating a healing diet, I think it is essential to get your digestive system back in excellent working order. And, in order to do that, I believe you must eliminate all food allergens and keep proteins and starches and proteins and fruit separate at every meal. But more about that later. After about three months of catering to your digestive system, the diet promoted by *The Zone* might be ideal. That will be for you to decide.

I relate all of this in the hope that you can learn more quickly than I did exactly what your body prefers. Don't get locked into a diet that isn't perfect for you by listening to anyone else, no matter what their credentials or the prevailing dietary dogma. As I'm sure you are aware, the government is now pushing a food pyramid with grains and starches as the base. They keep insisting that overweight America has to eat lots of starchy carbohydrates and almost no fat. If that works, why are our citizens getting heavier and heavier? Remember, cows are fed grains deliberately to *fatten* them! Although *saturated fat* is not health-promoting, there are other oils that are actually essential to good health. Essential fatty acids are critical to our well-being, and I fear a great many people are not getting them due to our public officials promoting dietary misinformation.

Most raw foods are easy to digest and cleansing, especially fruit. But staying with a raw food diet for very long left me weak and spacy. Whole grains contain lots of nutrients and are possibly an ideal food for some, but sticking to macrobiotics was not perfect for me. I lost all spontaneity, felt very dull and plodding, was frequently hungry and was having blood sugar highs and lows.

Since the very nature of food is so complex and the human race so diverse, how can anyone possibly figure out what constitutes a "perfect" diet, suitable for everyone? And how in the world can you know whom to trust and what to eat? I certainly don't have all the answers, and I'm not sure anyone else does. So, all of these conflicting opinions and complexities would really present you with a terrible dilemma if it weren't for one simple fact: YOUR BODY KNOWS.

Your cells not only communicate with each other, they would be most happy to communicate with you if you just let them. That is where paying attention and listening come in. YOU are the only person in this world who can determine exactly what you should eat.

You can get started on your own, individual path to true, energetic, exuberant health just by asking your body to assist you.

Keep in mind as you fine-tune your diet that your muscles, cells and immune system all need protein to rebuild. Also, that carbohydrates (which include *all* fruits, vegetables and grains) are converted to sugar before they are utilized by the body. The neutral vegetables and most fruits do not break down as quickly as the starches and are therefore, a better source of "slow release" sugar. Knowing these facts to start with should enable you to keep a steady supply of energy throughout the day and avoid the highs and lows so many of us have experienced.

Chapter Seventeen

———◆———

Alternative Options

Finding an open-minded doctor who does not restrict herself/himself to conventional or orthodox practices endorsed by the AMA is not always easy. They sometimes develop an attitude about the information they were given in medical school as being the only truth available. As you may remember, it was just a few short years ago that most of them declared that what you ate had nothing to do with the state of your health! They are not taught nutrition, so unless they have studied it on their own and have learned to recognize good food as one of the most powerful "medicines" on earth, they are not apt to endorse it as applicable in your case.

Many of them are still stuck in the treatment of symptoms rather than finding the cause of the problem and many are arrogant and negative about any alternative kinds of therapies and scoff at natural herbs or diet supplements. Some of them make a living operating — and sometimes operate too often.

On the other side of the coin, there are those who are sincerely searching for answers and open to new information. Some of the younger graduates, I am happy to say, seem to be less rigid and more open to alternative therapies. They blend their education with common sense, an open mind, and new studies to create true health practitioners. A really good doctor reminds me of my grandfather. He knows that he is not the healer but only the person who tries to assist the body in healing itself. As Hippocrates said, "The natural healing force within each one of us is the greatest force in getting well."

A quote from Thomas Edison just might be our insight into the possibilities to come. He said, "The doctor of the future will give no medicine but will interest his patients in the care of the human frame, in proper diet and in the cause and prevention of disease."

If you cannot find a satisfactory M.D., you might consider an alternative practitioner.

Homeopathy is based on the Law of Similars, which in essence states that like cures like. The founder, Samuel Hahnemann, maintained that symptoms are the body's defense mechanisms attempting to eliminate an illness. Effective medicines, he thought, produced a condition similar to the illness itself and therefore stimulated the immune system to more powerfully fight the disease. Homeopathy is similar to the approach taken by Hippocrates and Paracelsus. The royal family in Great Britain has used homeopathic medicine for many years.

Naturopathy is the use of many nontoxic, noninvasive healing methods. Its practitioners regard illness as the body's effort at self-cleansing and they believe that the underlying life force is the source of the body's ability to heal itself. Some of the most frequently used remedies to assist this life force are herbs. A healthful diet, elimination of toxins, good posture, and healthy emotions are all advocated by naturopathic doctors. They also employ quite a diverse combination of therapies including acupuncture, homeopathy, chiropractic, therapeutic massage, fasting, colonics, and hydrotherapy. They are well educated in the natural healing sciences and the accredited ones have attended a four-year program, learning most of the same information taught at conventional medical schools. They frequently prescribe vitamin and mineral supplements and, although they are committed to using nontoxic and noninvasive methods, they acknowledge that modern medical practices, such as surgery, have their place in crisis intervention.

It is my most fervent wish that every state in this union would allow the practice of naturopathy. That they are only permitted in eleven states to help our ailing citizens regain their health is, in my estimation, a sin against us all. We can, again, thank the AMA for pressuring state legislators to outlaw the practice of naturopathy. They were undoubtedly afraid (and for good reason) that informed and intelligent citizens might opt for naturopathic, preventative care instead of conventional reactive medicine.

Chiropractic is a method of treating disease based on the theory that disease is caused by interference with nerve function. Practitioners employ manipulation of the body joints, especially the spine, to try to restore normal nerve function. There are different methods of chiropractic manipulation, some being much more subtle and gentle than others.

Osteopathy is a school of medicine placing special emphasis on the interrelationship of the musculoskeletal system to all other body systems.

Acupuncture is the use of needles to direct qi energy (the Chinese name for life source pronounced "chee") to particular places in the body. The intent is to unblock the pathways, called meridians, to drain qi where it is excessive, to warm parts that are cool or stagnant, to reduce excessive heat, or to increase or decrease moisture. Acupuncture is only a small part of Chinese medicine, but it is the one most westerners have heard about. It has gained some popularity and recognition in this country mostly by people attempting to alleviate pain or needing assistance in overcoming addictions.

Most all of the medical sciences practiced now and throughout history (other than our own conventional, allopathic medicine) consider the symptoms of an illness only the indications of dysfunction or the attempt by the body to heal itself. They support or at least learn from the symptoms rather than attack them. My common sense tells me that modern medicine's habit of doing battle with the symptoms themselves has taken us in a most unhealthy direction.

In the Resources portion of this book, there are names of several medical associations that might be of help if you need them.

A relatively new book, *Dr. Rosenfeld's Guide to Alternative Medicine,* is an interesting discourse on methods of treatment other than those used by the "establishment." He tries to be unbiased and has made an attempt to find out what works and what doesn't.

However, Dr. Rosenfeld seems to have trouble with the word "toxins." He continually puts it in quotes as if there isn't really such a thing. At the same time he does not mention the incredible amount of toxic, chemical "nonfood" in our food supply, and I think every health practitioner in the country should be screaming about it!

Another doctor, Elson Haas, who has also written a book, considers detoxification the "missing link" in Western nutrition and a key to the health and vitality of our civilization.

So you see, you have to make decisions based on your own inner intelligence.

Dr. Rosenfeld also mentions a type of cancer, Hodgkin's disease, that according to him, can now almost always be cured by our conventional, chemical means, but does not give us any equally important information concerning the types of cancer that do *not* respond to conventional therapy. He does, however, admit that there is precious little in the form of effective treatment against advanced cancers.

He insists that naturopaths not be allowed to practice and his unwarranted and unexplained prejudice is quite a turn-off. He suggests that we check with the AMA to find out whether a therapy is valid or not. This is the same AMA that went to bed, politically, with the tobacco industry to oppose Medicare (with full knowledge of the terrible health hazards from tobacco), denied that they had, then recanted and admitted that, indeed, they had. I have lost all respect for the American Medical Association and wouldn't trust them with the health of my little finger. Their opinion, in my opinion, would be completely biased and totally unreliable and I am certainly not alone in this regard.

In spite of my criticisms, I think Dr. Rosenfeld's book is full of worthwhile information and quite interesting reading if you keep in mind that he is somewhat biased due to his education and his associations, even though he tries not to be.

My point is, we all have a tendency to believe everything that is in print, especially if it is written by someone with an M.D. or Ph.D behind their name. You can't afford to accept without question everything you read about conventional or alternative medicine. It may or may not be reliable information, and the author may have unreasonable prejudices. Trust your intuition, listen to your body and carefully research any therapy you intend to try.

Chapter Eighteen

———◆———

Reflexology and Other Safe Therapies

During the years of my "healing mode," I tried a number of things that may or may not have contributed to my recovery. I was always looking for possibilities that sounded reasonable, weren't costly or dangerous, but seemed to make sense. One such treatment was massaging the feet and applying pressure to the acupressure points diagrammed on reflexology charts.

I had also read somewhere that you could increase the circulation in your feet by immersing them in alternating baths of hot and cold water. Since both of my big toes were numb I figured they could use some attention so I started a nightly routine of first dipping them in and out of hot and cold water, then giving them a really intensive massage.

It not only made me feel that I was doing something positive to help my system heal itself, it felt wonderful. Just how much it contributed to my getting well, I couldn't say. However, I knew it couldn't hurt, it felt right, it felt good, it told my body that I was doing my utmost to assist it and therefore it was of value.

My point is, that there are a great many possibilities to be explored and investigated. Whether or not they have passed any scientific studies validating them in the eyes of those who care about such things is not an issue. The important thing to remember is to pay attention to your body's reaction to everything you try and make a note of it.

I had completely forgotten about my months of treating my feet until I had a restless, sleepless night not long ago. My legs and feet both seemed uneasy as I tossed and turned in bed. Finally, I paid attention, got out of bed, got some oil and gave my feet a wonderful rub down. I remember wondering, after I laid back down, if that would really help my insomnia. That's the last thing I remember until I woke up the next morning feeling very rested and refreshed. It worked very well indeed, because I paid attention to what was going on in my body.

Please don't try anything that might be detrimental or dangerous, but neither should you exclude anything just because someone else doesn't understand it. There are many options and disciplines that have been used by healers all over the world for many generations that may not make sense to our scientific culture. That makes them no less valid. Investigate. Learn all you can and try those that feel right. Always remember, it is your body, your responsibility and even your privilege to help it repair itself.

As I write this, some researchers are beginning to propose that bee venom can contribute to the control of M.S. Hurray, if it proves to be helpful!

I was introduced to the idea of bee venom therapy several years ago and chose to pursue the ideas described in this book rather than submit to a bunch of bees poking their sharp bottoms into my flesh.

I have no doubt, however, that there are other possibilities available. Just be cautious and investigate everything you try to make sure you don't make matters worse.

To me, the natural therapies are still a great deal safer than trying new drugs. Iatrogenic (doctor-caused) disease is a rapidly spreading epidemic. Infections acquired in hospitals, unnecessary operations resulting in needless deaths, side effects from dangerous drugs, health impairing X-rays and unnecessary medical treatment due to inaccurate lab reports are occurring in alarming numbers.

Some of the alternative therapies that seem to have healing potential are acupressure, acupuncture, aromatherapy, biofeedback training, breathwork, crystals, electromagnetism, flower remedies, guided imagery, hypnotherapy, light and color therapy, magnetic therapy, meditation, sound therapy and yoga. Don't dismiss any possibilities just because your doctor didn't study it in school. It has been my experience that several therapies I read about in new age and alternative-type publications several years ago are now being touted by the medical establishment.

Again, let me caution you not to try anything potentially dangerous, such as agreeing to submit to experimental chemotherapy! But keep an open mind, especially when it comes to therapies that bring up a very positive "yes" from your body. Things that stimulate and balance your body's subtle energy flow might be a great deal more healing than we realize.

Chapter Nineteen

◆

A Painful Lesson

A few years ago I was experimenting with tofu. I was trying to find some recipes using tofu that Art and I both liked. Several sounded really good, so for several nights in a row we ate tofu stuffed into this and that with tomato sauce poured liberally over each one. At that same time I was experiencing some pain in my left thumb joint, but in somewhat typical fashion, I chose to ignore it. (You would think I would learn!)

Suddenly, one morning, I awakened with an extremely painful shoulder which simply wouldn't cooperate when it came to fastening a bra or putting my arm up in the air. I mean, it was frozen!

The acupuncturist was my first thought, so I went straight to his office. I eventually had four treatments. Each one helped for a few hours and then the stiffness and the pain returned. (I was still experimenting with the tofu-tomato sauce recipes.) It became obvious that needles weren't the answer so I returned to my many volumes on food and healing.

The answer, it turned out, was a family of plants called nightshades. It seems that many people are sensitive to the nightshade family to one degree or another. Some people can't eat them at all without suffering, some have to overdo it, as I did, to become arthritic, and then some people aren't bothered at all. The nightshades include tomatoes, potatoes, eggplant, peppers and tobacco.

As soon as I read about them I realized what I had done with all that tomato sauce. I immediately started avoiding cooked tomatoes, went back for one more acupuncture treatment, and haven't had any trouble since. Art and I are both, we discovered, fairly sensitive to the nightshades. We don't have to avoid them completely, but when our joints start twinging we know we've had too many. Cooked tomatoes are quite acidic, so use them cautiously.

Some people who suffer from arthritis are not only quite sensitive to the nightshades, but also have difficulty with fruit, especially citrus. Because we are all so different, the only way to know about yourself is to "ask" your body.

Because cooked tomatoes are so acidic, I decided that decreasing my intake of all acidic foods and increasing the alkaline foods as well as avoiding nightshades might make my joints feel lubricated and pain free. Sure enough, for me it works. I have no scientific studies at my disposal to verify that it works for anyone else but it is something you might try if you suffer from painful joints. Three very alkalizing foods are vegetable broth, watermelon, and the oriental umeboshi plum.

If you wake up in the morning with a sour taste in your mouth, chances are you should incorporate more alkaline foods in your diet.

Chapter Twenty

———◆———

Let Food Be Your Medicine

It might help you a great deal if you take that statement by Hippocrates quite literally: "Let food be your medicine" should mean exactly that. Instead of feeling deprived you can look at every bit of food, for a while, just as you would look at a prescription. (And food is a whole lot more palatable!)

To a pill-popping society, an apple may appear to be an innocuous thing, but to most bodies it is manna from heaven. Once you have discovered what your particular body likes and dislikes, *treat it to the most powerful and effective medicine on earth:* the food it needs to heal itself.

If you are taking any prescribed medicine, keep your doctor informed, for as you start the healing process your need for pharmaceutical props will begin to disappear. Therefore, your doctor will need to adjust the dosage until you no longer need it at all. I sincerely hope that you have a health practitioner instead of a pill pusher. If so, the healthier you get and the less medicine you need, the more you will be encouraged to continue on your path. If the opposite is true, I would hope that you have the determination to find another doctor.

I go to a young medical doctor who says that he's not really holistic, but he does accept my method and my opinions about my health as valid. He is there for me in emergencies and cares that I am healthy no matter how I choose to get there. I can ask no more from someone who was trained to write prescriptions.

So, be positive about the changes in your diet. When the lack of sugar and saturated fat is noticeable compared to what you are used to eating, simply look at the food on your plate as a bunch of healing energy your system can hardly wait to utilize, because that's exactly what it is.

It is really amazing to me that my taste in food has changed so much over the years. A great many things I used to eat quite frequently are no longer the least bit appealing. It is very much like giving up smoking. For a while you love the smell of cigarette smoke and are constantly thinking about having deprived yourself of such a pleasure only to find, down the road, that the smoke is not at all pleasant and you can't imagine how you used to enjoy pulling that horrible stuff into your lungs!

Let food be your medicine and you will eventually find that you don't need any other kind.

I don't mean to suggest that changing your way of eating is easy. We have established our social interaction around the dinner table. Friends and relatives are not always supportive of what they consider a strange diet. I learned a long time ago to say as little as possible about what I planned to eat when out for a social evening. Most of my friends know what I eat and what I don't eat, so they are more apt to ask if a restaurant they suggest has enough on the menu to accommodate me.

When we are going to a large party and I am quite certain there won't be much there for me to eat I will eat something before we go or take a small snack with me.

My greatest accomplishment when cooking for others came about just a few years ago at Thanksgiving. My oldest daughter, her husband, and their three teen-age children were coming to visit even though I had stated that I planned on serving a turkeyless meal. I carefully planned the menu to include foods I knew they liked and included some, such as stuffed squash that they had never eaten. Even the teenagers were more than happy with the selection and were full of praise for "Mimi's" food. They later confessed that their mother had cooked them a turkey before they came, but that my dinner was just as good. I wouldn't have believed them if I hadn't seen them eat with such enthusiasm.

Chapter Twenty-one

◆

Caffeine, Coffee, Colas and Chocolate

Caffeine, which is a methyixanthine DRUG is a stimulant to the central nervous system. It increases your heart rate, blood pressure and stomach acid among other unhealthy effects. Anyone concerned about osteoporosis should know that because caffeine increases the acid in your system, your body will remove calcium from your bones to protect the pH balance in your blood. It is also a diuretic, which reduces the amount of many vitamins and minerals in your body.

Add these concerns to the fact that toxic chemicals are used in commercial coffee production, both regular and decaf, and you should have plenty of reasons to switch to something more compatible with optimum health.

Soft drinks containing caffeine are certainly no better. They are either loaded with sugar or contain an artificial sweetener. "Artificial" anything is not food. The fact is, aspartame is made using genetic biotechnology and is potentially dangerous. Also, cola drinks get their brown color from a compound that is certainly not a health food.

Chocoholics are, as the name implies, addicted to choco-late. They are addicted because of the caffeine content which stimulates the adrenal glands again and again until they are ex-hausted and can do no more. Chocolate is also hard on your liver. A little chocolate is no big deal to a healthy body, but if you have less than optimum health, it is an unnecessary aggravation.

The human body likes to feel good. That's natural. But what we have done is replace real, continuous health and energy with artificial stimulants which keep us from experiencing the real thing.

Of course they are hard to give up. They are addictive! But as long as you continue to use them you are depriving your-self of any chance to become truly energetic and vibrantly alive. Since many people have not felt vibrant for a long time, they have forgotten what it feels like and what they are missing. How very sad.

A healing diet is far from addictive. You might even feel worse before you get better because if you are loaded with tox-ins, they are going to get stirred up as your body starts getting rid of them. You will probably have headaches if you go through caffeine withdrawal. I can only promise you that it is ultimately worth every bit of discomfort to enjoy the energy you will expe-rience in a very short time.

Another big problem in our food supply is cow's milk. Now that they have removed the fat in skim milk, all that's left are the two troublemakers: lactose and milk protein. Most adults have difficulty digesting lactose, so when it gets to the colon bac-teria ferment it, converting it to gas and lactic acid. The allergic reaction people have to milk comes from the antibody reaction to its proteins. Antibodies are formed in the blood stream as a reac-tion to something the body recognizes as foreign. They can raise havoc every time that substance is ingested. Milk allergy can cause chronic diarrhea, urticaria, eczema or atopic dermatitis.

There is also scientific data that suggests the antibodies are connected to rheumatoid arthritis and diabetes and that ho-mogenization might play a role in heart disease. The high heat of pasteurization denatures any of milk's food value and, along with homogenization, increases its indigestibility.

When you consider all of this, then add the use of recombinant bovine growth hormone and preservatives and the unavoidable pesticide residue, you have a very questionable "healthy food"!

I wish all those celebrities would wipe the milk mustaches off their faces and learn a few pertinent facts about the product they tout so joyfully.

Chapter Twenty-two

◆

Healthful Substitutes

Most of the ingredients listed below are available at natural, health food stores. If there isn't one near you, look in the back of the book under resources. You can get most anything by mail order.

Coffee — Try instant, roasted, grain beverages such as Pero and Kaffree Roma. Teccino is a tasty one (of different flavors) you brew in your coffee appliance. Some coffee substitutes are in tea bags.

Tea — There are a great many delicious herb teas. Try several. Most are good both hot and cold. Green tea is a super antioxidant but the flavor isn't to my liking.

Sugar — Honey and maple syrup are the ones most commonly used, but although they are natural, they are still simple sugars that should be used sparingly. Other substitutes are brown rice syrup and barley malt syrup. Both are complex carbohydrates that enter the blood stream more slowly. Stevia is the sweet herb I mentioned that you can use, but be careful as it is VERY sweet. To use stevia, you dissolve the white powder in pure water and measure it in drops. It will keep indefinitely in the refrigerator. Fruit juices and dried fruit are other possibilities for incorporating a sweet taste in cooking.

Chocolate — Carob can be substituted for cocoa (in equal amounts), but I like to add a little roasted grain powder also, for a richer flavor. Even then, it still will never taste like chocolate!

Colas — There are a great many bottled drinks in health food stores to choose from, but they all contain too much sugar in one form or another. Try making your own herb tea and adding a drop of stevia if you must have something sweet to drink. If you consume lots of pure water every day, you won't crave other liquids so much.

Fats and oils — Do not use hydrogenated or partially hydrogenated oils such as margarine (and they are abundant in manufactured grocery items) or highly refined polyunsaturated oils such as safflower, sunflower or corn. Ideally, you should get a mixture of different high-quality, unaltered fats in your diet. Use fresh, cold-processed polyunsaturated oils like sesame, canola and grapeseed oil and monounsaturated oils like extra virgin olive oil. Very limited amounts of saturated fat like butter (especially ghee, which is butter without the milk solids) and fresh coconut (which yields about a tablespoon of oil per ounce of coconut) are much better for you than any of the oils man has fooled with. Sesame oil has a nice flavor for oriental dishes and a small amount of the dark, roasted sesame oil added to another oil makes an oriental salad taste authentic. Just keep in mind that anything refined such as flour, sugar or oil has literally had the life taken out of it, so it is actually a nonfood. The bugs have sense enough not to eat it so why should you?

Milk — There are several healthful substitutes for milk. If your meal is a starch meal you can use rice milk or oat milk. My preference is oat milk, but either will work. You can find them both at health food stores or by mail order. For a protein meal there are even more substitutes: soy milk, tofu milk, almond or cashew milk. Soy milk is hard for me to digest, so I simply put silken tofu in a blender with water and make a smooth, easy to digest milk for cooking. Blanched almonds blended with water and strained, or raw cashews blended with water make delicious milks for "cream" sauces, gravies, or soups. You can also cream soups for starch meals with potatoes, cooked barley, oats or rice.

To make the nut milks, you simply put a third to a half of a cup of blanched almonds or raw cashews in a blender with one cup of water and blend until very smooth, then add one more cup of water and blend again. (The amount of nuts depends on how rich you want it.) Strain the almond milk through a fine strainer.

Agar-agar — This is a sea vegetable that is flavorless and makes a good substitute for gelatin (which is produced by very unappetizing means).

Arrowroot or Kudzu — Both are natural thickeners and are good replacements for corn starch or flour, which turn quickly to sugar in your body.

Chapter Twenty-three

◆

The Great Debate About Losing Weight

How many diet books do you suppose have been written? We are constantly bombarded with news about studies on obesity, what's to blame and how to fix it. Almost every day a very fat rat and a thin rat are on public view with the latest theory on weight gain. Millions of people have lost the same ten or more pounds over and over again, only to end up heavier than when they started.

If, in order to regain your health, you are eating the kinds of food your body likes, combining it properly, and not overeating, you will automatically lose weight — unless you are underweight, in which case you will probably gain. You see, a truly healthy body knows exactly what it should weigh, and it will see to it that you get there if you give it a chance.

I am talking about eating a balanced diet and eating only until you are satisfied and not until you feel full.

Most of us have mistreated our digestive systems for so long that they will take a while to recover. A good digestive aid and a good attitude will go a long way in your battle over the bulge. I'm not suggesting that you concern yourself with or concentrate on losing weight. I'm talking about you being the healthiest that you can possibly be, given your genetics and taking into account any irreversible organ damage.

I'm also talking about quality of life. Good health is something most of us take for granted until we lose it. Going on one diet after another and rebounding into fat city is a good way to compromise one's health.

Pursue only one goal, good health, and all the weight that should come off will come off. What have you got to lose, except those extra pounds and your annoying or painful symptoms?

Fruits and vegetables are full of fiber, vitamins, minerals, phytochemicals and subtle energy. They generate a powerful biochemical, hormonal response by your body which cannot be duplicated by drugs.

Please don't fall for diet pills or any other unnatural methods of losing weight. Just use food as your medicine!

Chapter Twenty-four

———◆———

Your Digestive System

A tremendous number of adverse physical conditions will respond positively when you activate the healing process by respecting and repairing your digestive system.

People don't usually attribute allergies, arthritis, rashes and other, more serious diseases to their eating habits and the subsequent stomach malfunction. But the chain reaction and downward spiral to ill health is first set in motion by incomplete digestion and assimilation.

Relating all of the processes involved in digesting and assimilating vital nutrients would require a whole, separate book, but here are some of the basics.

The lack of stomach vitality and digestive juices creates a problem for all the other organs involved in digestion, from the pancreas to the liver. Harmful bacteria are not destroyed, beneficial intestinal flora are overwhelmed by pathogenic microorganisms which excrete over seventy different kinds of toxins into your system.

The liver, which has some five hundred known physical functions, becomes overloaded and incapable of cleansing the blood completely. An inefficient liver can create such diverse conditions as hormonal imbalance, fatigue, underactive thyroid, moodiness, hemorrhoids, blood sugar problems and high blood-fat levels. Medical tests to ascertain the condition of the liver only show a problem *after* the liver cells have ruptured, spilling their enzymes into the blood stream. By then, every cell in the body has been subjected to irritants in the blood stream for a long time.

The gallbladder also becomes sluggish and toxic, creating more health problems, and the kidneys are asked to filter things they weren't designed to filter, which increases their load and interferes with their normal functions.

The vicious cycle continues with ever increasing vitamin and mineral deficiencies, more and more toxins in the blood stream, slower and slower digestion by irritated organs, leading to more fermentation, and more liver overload.

This is an extremely simplified explanation of a most complex process, but I'm sure you get the idea.

Eventually the lymph system becomes upset with so much extra waste to eliminate, and when that happens the immune system gets involved and becomes overactive, underactive or confused.

And it all starts when you chew your food.

Don't think that just because you don't have an upset stomach frequently that you don't have a problem with digestion. If you have any sign of ill health you had better start paying strict attention to this most important process and clean up your diet and your eating habits.

You actually aren't what you eat, you are what you eat *that is digested properly.* Your system is crippled by food that is not completely digested. One path leads to vibrant health and the other to disease.

Our mothers were right. We need to do a better job of chewing our food! Our society is certainly on the fast track. We don't just eat fast foods, we gobble them down. This leads to so much indigestion that the Tums-type manufacturers are making a killing off of our slow demise. The reason we should carefully chew our food is that our initial ability to digest takes place in the mouth. That is why we have teeth and saliva. No matter what the quality of the food you consume, if you don't chew it into a liquid before you swallow it you aren't going to reap all the benefits from it. And it certainly isn't conducive to good digestion to have your stomach bombed by giant food particles.

When you overeat, you get the same result: stomach mistreatment. (If you take time to really chew your food your jaw gets too tired to allow you to overeat). These two factors, chewing thoroughly and, as a consequence, eating moderately, could be the diet to end all diets. We could call it the "Tired Jaw Diet," write a book and make a fortune.

I challenge you to eat your next meal with careful attention to the number of times you chew each bite before you swallow. For your health's sake, you should chew between twenty-five and fifty times, depending on the size of the bite and the type of food. If you're not even coming close, consider the stress and toxins you are creating and the energy you are wasting trying to digest food in chunks.

When it comes to digestion, some foods are easy and some are not. The quality and purity of the food is important, and how you combine foods can make a big difference.

Keep it simple. If you are in ill health at the present time, your top priority should be simply to get well. After you have nurtured your body back to health, you can investigate all the great recipes and gourmet health foods that await your pleasure. Don't give in to a feeling of deprivation and self-pity because you can't eat what the people around you are eating. Look at it as a learning experience, a gustatory adventure, a fabulous new diet, a spiritual experience, or whatever attitude you need to take to keep yourself in a healing mode. Remember, attitude is extremely important.

Try to find a source for organic fresh fruits and vegetables. They may cost a little more, but the taste, lack of toxins and increased nutrients are more than worth the added expense.

Regular supermarkets are beginning to carry some organic produce. If yours is not, urge the manager to start. Call around and see if any farmers in your area are farming organically, or grow some of your own, using pots, if necessary. If you don't have a local source for the other organic foods I suggest, there is a list of mail order sources in the back of this book.

Always carry your digestive enzymes with you when eating out and chew a few after dining. If you consume fried foods (which is not really a good choice in a healing diet), it is a good idea to ask for some horseradish, as it will help with the digestion of fat.

Trust yourself and take charge of your health. No one else is going to do it for you because they can't. If you are the least bit patient, you will notice an improvement of some kind very quickly. Note each positive feeling in your diary and you'll eventually have a number of milestones you can look back on with satisfaction and pride. Above all, don't let anyone talk you out of your program with negative words of discouragement. It is your life, your body, your health and your responsibility. I can't begin to count the number of people with medical degrees who have insisted, or at least inferred, that my symptoms simply disappeared of their own accord. Let me guarantee you, they did not! I would stake my life on it! Just remember my diary and the cause and effect connection between my food intake and my symptoms.

Please don't give in to feelings of self-pity and decide this is your fate. As long as we live we can make choices about our future. If you sit down and give up, you might find it pleasant for a while, being waited on and catered to. But you will sacrifice so much quality of life and end up completely helpless sometime down the road. Take charge of your life by taking care of your stomach!

Chapter Twenty-five

◆

The Remarkable Story of Charles Benge

My friend Charlie, from Houston, who is now seventy-two years young, was first diagnosed with prostate cancer in February of 1990. His urologist performed surgery (implanting gold seeds) in March. He then had Charlie undergo radiation for five weeks. "That really knocked out my immune system," Charlie tells me.

Every six months he reported back to the urologist. Every other trip they did a bone scan and the other times they did a blood test.

In 1995, the test for Charlie's PSA (Prostate Specific Antigen) started rising again but his urologist assured him it was nothing to be concerned about. This went on for two years with the PSA steadily rising two or three points every six months and the urologist still unconcerned.

In January 1997, Charlie had his regular physical exam by his general practitioner who stated, "You are beginning to have a problem." His PSA was then 9.7. The doctor sent him back to the urologist for blood work. When the lab report came back, an assistant to the urologist told Charlie his PSA was 14.0

and they wanted to start him on hormones. "No sir, not today," stated Charlie and he walked out.

One month later Charlie was at the M.D. Anderson Hospital in Houston and his PSA was 17.0. They performed a biopsy which came back positive.

"They recommended radical surgery," says Charlie, "and wanted to put a tube out my side with a flap on it. I declined that invitation and asked what else could be done."

"You could be castrated," offered the doctor.

Charlie declined that also and asked for another alternative.

"Hormones," the doctor replied.

"That's just chemical castration," said Charlie. "What happens if I don't do any of those things?"

"Then you are going to die," the doctor declared.

Charlie said he would make a judgement about all that later and left M.D. Anderson.

Charlie and his wife, Midge, immediately contacted "People Against Cancer" who took his medical records and sent them to doctors all over the world. They eventually recommended a doctor in Michigan who put Charlie on a regimen that included a diet of organic food, supplements, digestive system support and herbs. He started the program October 16, 1997.

"It requires discipline," says Charlie, "but I am sticking with it." In December, his doctor, the general practitioner, reported that his PSA was down to 8.7. In February they did a complete blood test and not only was his PSA 2.5 (anything below 3.0 is considered normal) but all of his seventy-two-year-old organs appeared to be functioning perfectly!

Charlie is aiming for a PSA of .1 which is considered "cured." He is then taking the test results back to the previously unconcerned urologist. (And knowing Charlie, he might have a few choice words to say.)

One of the most remarkable things about this story is the reaction of some of Charlie's golfing friends who are doctors. When he tells them the details of his PSA improvement, their reply is simply "I don't believe it." What an easy way for them to close their minds! They don't have to question their belief systems, their prejudices, or their lack of knowledge about nutrition. " I don't believe it" leaves them free to discount the possibility of curing the incurable.

Charlie's doctor in Michigan told him that he no longer practices medicine, he now practices nutrition. He also believes that proper digestion is the key to good health. That's two of us among a growing number of others.

Long live Charlie!

The phone number for "People Against Cancer" is: 515/972-4444.
Email: nocancer@ix.netcom.com
Web Site: HTTP:\\www.dodgenet.com\nocancer

Chapter Twenty-six

◆

Combining Foods

W hen you first start the follow-
ing regimen, it may seem rather restrictive. But I would guess
that self-indulgence or carelessness got you where you are today
and it is time to pay your dues. If you follow this program for
just three weeks, you will notice a big difference in the way you
feel. Your energy level will rise dramatically, any chronic aches
and pains will diminish and your overall sense of well being will
increase. After that, if you will stick with it for about three months,
you will have your digestive system in shape to handle a less
strict diet. Just remember, no matter what you put in your mouth,
chew, chew, chew.

1. Don't eat proteins and starchy carbohydrates at
the same meal. It takes two different digestive juices for these
foods. One is acid and the other one alkaline. They have a tendency to cancel each other out, which leaves you with poorly
digested food. You can, however, enjoy a long list of nonstarchy
vegetables with your protein and these same wonder foods, known
as neutrals can be combined with the starches with no problem.

The starchy foods are all the grains and products made
from them, such as bread and crackers. The starchy vegetables
are all the dry beans, corn, lentils, parsnips, potatoes (both sweet
and white), pumpkin, winter squash and Jerusalem artichokes.

Dried, split peas are starchy but fresh green ones are not. If you get confused and you don't have a list in front of you, you are pretty safe if the color of the vegetable you want to eat with your protein is green or red. The starchy ones are mostly orange, brown or white. The protein, or building foods, are all meats, fish, dairy, eggs, nuts, nut butters and soy foods.

2. Do not eat sweets and protein at the same meal. This is the worst combination for healthful digestion.

3. Do not eat fruits, raw or cooked, and protein at the same meal.

4. It is best to eat raw fruits by themselves because they will digest alone in about an hour and if you combine them with anything else their digestion will be delayed and they will start to ferment. A byproduct of fermentation is gas. Use raw fruits as snacks between meals and try to eat plenty of them. Cooked fruits, for most people, will combine just fine with the starches.

Any vegetable not mentioned under starches is neutral, as are mushrooms and raw tomatoes.

You will find a list of all these foods in the recipe section of this book. To make it as easy as possible for you to learn this discipline, I have organized the recipe section, into protein (Acid), starch (Alkaline) or vegetable (Neutral).

* Neutrals can be combined with either acid (protein) or alkaline (starch).

* Put together as many neutrals and alkalines or neutrals and acids as you like.

* Eat three protein-neutral meals a day or, at least, two protein-neutral meals and one starch-neutral meal. The neutrals are the nutrient rich, healing wonder foods, so try to emphasize your intake of them.

You will find that you can put really great meals together following this discipline. For example, for a protein-neutral meal you might have a soup creamed with tofu or almond milk, a large green salad sprinkled with walnuts or pecans, a piece of broiled fish and a sizeable serving of mixed vegetables. For a starch-neutral meal you could choose the baked potato soup, a vegetable salad and beans with brown rice.

Snack on fruit, raw vegetables, and very occasionally, sweets without refined sugar. Just make sure the sweets don't cross the line by containing protein.

Avoid refined sugar as if it were arsenic. It is a terrible thing to eat.

I am really not fond of cooking and never have been. Most of the recipes I use are fairly quick and easy because there are other things I'd rather do. Raw foods, which are cleansing, full of nutrients and enzymes, and easy to digest are the quickest and easiest!

Chapter Twenty-seven

---◆---

The Fastest, Shortest Path Is the Best!

How often in your life have you been told that the longest, hardest way to do something was the best? It seemed to me, growing up, that every time I tried to take a shortcut in doing or learning, I was told that the better way was the longer way.

I have good news. Of all the disciplines I tried in my search for health, this way of eating is the one that rewarded me the fastest and the most.

It is fairly difficult to find recipes that adhere to the idea that proteins and starches or proteins and sweets should not be eaten together. That is due, in part, because many people don't know it makes digestion more difficult. Another reason is that people with perfectly healthy, efficient digestive systems can handle these combinations (but only to a certain degree and only people with strong, young digestive systems.)

Since we are talking about using food as medicine, we need a way of eating that gives your body the most nutrients for the least effort, one that allows your system to get rid of stored toxins, eventually purifies and nourishes every cell, and promotes the body's programmed healing capacity.

I have read articles by experts who say it doesn't matter how you combine the food you eat. My answer is, TRY IT. If it doesn't make a difference, you'll know it very quickly. If it does, you'll know the truth because it works!

Due to this way of combining food, I no longer have to battle candida, I have more energy, my arthritic symptoms have disappeared, my overall sense of well-being is greater, and my legs are stronger than ever.

Since I am not a gourmet cook or a purist about ingredients, I often use minced garlic in a jar, dried onion flakes, canned beans (organic, with no sugar added), and anything else that makes cooking easier and faster. Because I use fresh, organic vegetables and fruit, these dishes still contain the nutrients necessary for health. I also cook with wine. It adds so much flavor to some dishes and if the food doesn't taste good, no matter how good it might be for us, we won't eat it.

My main objective was to create quick, simple recipes that would give you the incentive to eat more of the things you should be eating and make them taste good.

An ideal diet and way of eating is going to be abandoned if it is too difficult, too complex or too bland, or all of the above. I know many people don't have the time or interest in spending hours in the kitchen, so many of the recipes are completed in just a few minutes.

I often use a food processor. I bought a little tiny one and keep it out where I use it. It handles most everything in one or two batches and is very simple to use and to clean.

Please don't get the impression that I always eat the right foods and deny myself all sensual enjoyment and the wicked delight that we humans seem to share when we disobey what we know to be the "right thing to do."

When I was really intent on getting well, I was much more disciplined than I am now because I knew if I veered off the path, I would immediately suffer the consequences. Now it takes a great deal more "veering" to notice a weakening or unusual fatigue.

Actually, I am usually pretty good about staying on track, because the slightest hint of a symptom raising its ugly head is too frightening to ignore. But I do enjoy my life completely and am well aware of my limits — a far cry from the depressed, exhausted, crippled and confused patient of 15 years ago.

In the past few years, I have become a great deal more healthy than many of my friends by using natural remedies and whole, unpolluted foods. Most of them take pain-killers, tranquilizers, diuretics, high blood pressure medicine or artificial drugs for arthritis, and they suffer from high cholesterol, blocked arteries, indigestion, irritable bowel syndrome, diverticulosis and many other deplorable conditions due mostly to their diet. The sad fact is that most of their medicines are affecting them as negatively as their diets.

It is such a shame that most people don't give any consideration to changing their diets until a real disaster strikes. I know I didn't. They will put up with less than optimal health, probably out of ignorance more than anything else. They also don't give much thought to all the side effects of drugs because they don't know they have an option.

If you have read this far, you have reason to rejoice. There are options and there are alternatives. There is hope and there is better health at your disposal. It is up to you.

Chapter Twenty-eight

◆

A Program for Whatever Ails You

So far, I've only talked about multiple sclerosis and candida because those were my battles. The fact is, a great many people in this country and elsewhere, with a great variety of diseases, have taken responsibility for their own health and have assisted their bodies in becoming vibrant and wholesome. It doesn't happen overnight and sometimes there are discouraging setbacks, but those who persevere are rewarded with an energy and enthusiasm for living that can hardly be described. Just think, it could be you!

Here, then, is a way of attacking the problem of ill health, no matter what the diagnosis.

1. Start your diary. Again, let me stress how important this is. Get a notebook and spend some time recording the date, how you are feeling (in detail), and what your doctor has had to say about it. Note also the kinds of foods you are eating. Include anything else that your intuition tells you might be pertinent, such as possible environmental pollutants, hereditary factors, family histories, etc. Discipline yourself to keep this record daily until you have regained your health or you are at least positive you are on the right path. If you will be fairly precise about your daily diet and activities, as well as how you are feeling each day, you will begin to interpret your body's messages more easily and

start to see patterns emerging that will help you determine what works and what doesn't.

2. *Discover your allergies* and clean up your diet. This applies to everyone, not just those with autoimmune diseases. Consider the fact that a body already stressed with a malfunction is doubly stressed when it has to cope with something it perceives as a foreign enemy, an allergen. You don't need but one battle to fight!

You don't have to accept any one discipline on diet such as raw foods or macrobiotics. Develop your own. But the basis for all healthful diets is the same: whole, unadulterated, unprocessed, unrefined, preferably organic, uncontaminated food. Eat in the manner I described — no protein and starch together, etc.— to get your digestive system back to an efficient, health-producing state. If you get hungry between meals eat fresh fruit or raw vegetables.

You will find, as you switch to wholesome foods, that your taste begins to change and you are able to easily consume the five fruits and/or vegetables that our government now, I'm happy to say, recommends. Remember the saying "An apple a day keeps the doctor away"? Old adages such as that survive because they contain truths we often, sadly, ignore.

3. Start reading everything you can find about your particular problem and how others have dealt with it. Note in your diary any solutions you want to try.

You will find, in the back this book, a number of books I recommend that you read. It is, by no means, a complete list of helpful information, but they are ones that most enlightened and educated me in the field of nutrition, diet and health.

4. Recruit your mind in a big way. Use your imagination to picture the healing processes you desire. Meditate by focusing on different parts of your body and silently inquire what is wrong and what you can do to help. Don't be surprised if you start receiving some very clear answers.

Learn about self-hypnosis and make yourself a tape. Play it to yourself at every opportunity.

Remember that your subconscious truly believes and acts on the things you repeatedly think and say about yourself. When people ask you how you are, you have three choices to make in your reply: "Oh, about the same" or "I'm really sick and getting worse" or "I am getting healthier and stronger every day." Since you are going to convince your subconscious with the repetition of one of these options, which one do you prefer?

Get an attitude! Don't let anyone discourage you.

5. Exercise a little each day, if at all possible. Our bodies were designed to function better with movement. You breathe deeper, release stress, and unblock channels for energy as well as promote the release of toxins with exercise. If you can't walk perhaps you can swim. Tai Chi movements are an excellent way to tone muscles and improve your health. It took me a long time to hold any Tai Chi posture, but the trying itself was worthwhile and eventually I could do it. A real milestone!

6. Purify your water or drink pure bottled water. The Centers for Disease Control estimate that over 1,000 people in this country will die each year from "approved" drinking water that has become tainted. Another 400,000 to as many as 27 MILLION people are expected to become ill from drinking contaminated water! The EPA's guidelines allow for "acceptable" amounts of chemicals such as chlorine byproducts, lead, arsenic, aluminum and dozens of other toxins in your drinking water, and even those standards aren't being met in many cases. If you are trying to overcome an illness, it is imperative that your body doesn't have to deal with more toxins from fecal matter, pesticides and virulent strains of parasites now finding their way into our drinking water. Fluoride is another toxic metal implicated in the development of M.S. Get rid of it in your drinking water and find a toothpaste that doesn't contain it.

7. Scrub your skin often with a loofa or a dry brush to remove dead layers of skin. The largest organ you possess for eliminating toxins is your skin, and it is much harder to eliminate toxins if your pores are plugged. The medical community keeps blaming the sun and a hole in the ozone layer for the increase in

skin cancer, but they need to take a good, hard look at the polluted food supply and the tremendous amount of nonfoods our bodies have to eliminate. Perhaps toxins plus skin plus sun equals a lot of skin cancer?

8. Take some kind of probiotic. Probiotics (meaning "for life" as opposed to antibiotic, "against life") are the friendly microorganisms that should be residing in your intestinal tract. You are probably in short supply due to antibiotics, chlorine, stress and too much sugar. These friendly microorganisms are an *essential* element in getting your body back to health. They help guard your body against harmful bacteria, yeast and viruses, produce essential vitamins, maintain your chemical and hormonal balance, counteract cancer-causing compounds in the colon, and perform a vast number of tasks for maintaining high energy levels and proper immune function. Lactobacillus acidophilus is one common probiotic supplement found in health food stores, but I take a supplement that contains several kinds of resident as well as transient microorganisms. You will find it listed in the Resources section of this book. This is one of those alternative medical therapies that I feel will be embraced by the conventional medical community in the near future. If so, it will enhance the health of millions as they become aware of its potential.

9. Try the supplements I mentioned in Chapter 15. I especially urge you to take some kind of chlorophyll in addition to the vitamins and minerals.

10. Be aware of abnormal gravitational fields, such as electric blankets, and avoid them whenever possible. These fields generate power at frequencies out of sync with the body's own electrical rhythms.

This is a relatively new science having to do with the magnetic and electrical systems within the body. We are exposed to so many "positive" fields such as microwave ovens, electric clocks, and other electrical appliances, that the earth's "negative" or health-producing fields around us are getting out of balance. Someone sitting in front of a computer every day needs to study this phenomenon and perhaps shield themselves from this constant exposure. Something else worth studying.

11. Find a doctor that has an open mind. It is getting easier now because some of them have started questioning the close-minded attitude of the AMA. You may have decided that I don't like doctors. Not true. I only dislike those who think that M.D. stands for Medical Deity. A really good doctor is a treasure. There are also the alternative practitioners that you might consider.

12. Be patient. This is the hard one. As I said before, healing from the inside out takes time. After years of neglect and mistreatment, your miraculous system is in disrepair. Clean it out, fuel it up with good nutrition, and give it time to heal itself. They say that we are never static. That is, we are either getting better or we are getting worse. As long as you feel that your symptoms are not getting worse, be enthusiastically optimistic. If you are not getting worse, you must be getting better!

13. You also need to keep an open mind. Things that I originally decided were "New Age" nonsense have since been proven to be quite effective. For instance, the use of essential oils (which were actually used in early Egypt) are becoming another arsenal in the natural therapy movement. Use your common sense but don't eliminate any of your options without investigation.

14. Be thankful. Sometimes when you're feeling rotten this is not easy, but nothing lifts our spirits more than counting our blessings and being grateful for the things we have. If you will look at your illness as one of life's learning experiences, you may even be grateful someday that you had to go through it. I know I now have more compassion, more gratitude, more knowledge, and more understanding than I did before. I also have my priorities in better order.

15. Consider a cleansing diet. Internal cleansing by way of fasting used to be a safe way to help the body get rid of toxins. However, there are now far too many environmental poisons that can cause toxic overload and your liver can easily become

overwhelmed trying to get rid of them. Dr. Elson Haas has written a comprehensive book on the subject called *The Detox Diet*. Don't go on any kind of detoxification program without knowing what the dangers as well as the benefits might be. One possibility is a one-day-a-week fast, when you ingest nothing but healthful liquids. This is one way of helping your digestive system by letting it rest and recuperate one day a week. It is also a relatively safe way to go because it doesn't overwhelm your liver.

16. Dare to question authorities. The history of mankind is full of examples of "the establishment" hounding and even crucifying those who made new discoveries that disagreed with conventional thought. Remember the ridicule endured by the men who proposed that the sun did not revolve around the earth; the earth was not flat; man could fly; vitamin C might help alleviate symptoms of the common cold; and what you eat might affect the state of your health. Do you recall that, many years ago, when it was suggested that physicians wash their hands before operating, they threw a fit?! There will always be those who defend the status quo and those who dare to question ridiculous logic. Dare to question and dare to trust your intuitive, inner wisdom in spite of the scorn of the "great white-coated ones" It's YOUR life and YOUR health at stake.

If this seems a bit overwhelming, please note that you aren't going to have to do it all at once. Some may dive right in to the whole program and some may take it a small step at a time. The first two are the really important steps that must be implemented in the beginning and continued as long as you have any health problems. The others are important, but can be stretched out over a period of time. Take it at your own pace, but try them all. I know the results will be worth the effort.

Chapter Twenty-nine

◆

Familiar and Unfamiliar Ingredients

S ome of the foods and flavorings I use may be items with which you are not familiar. Others may be old friends. Please try the new ones. You just might love them.

Aduki Beans — (sometimes Adzuki) a small, dark red bean used in macrobiotic cooking. Cooks quickly without soaking.

Agar-agar — A gelatinous seaweed that replaces gelatin. It is more nutritious and gels more easily.

Almond Milk — (and Almond cream) – For milk, blend 1/3 cup of blanched almonds with 1 cup of water until smooth. Add 1 more cup of water and blend. Strain through a fine sieve. For cream, blend 1/2 cup of blanched almonds with 1 cup of water and strain through a fine sieve.

Arrowroot — A white herbal powder used to thicken sauces and gravies. It replaces flour and cornstarch.

Balsamic vinegar — A delicious, sweet vinegar made from grapes. It is aged in a different kind of wooden cask each year and is marvelous in salad dressings. Buy one of the better ones, because a little goes a long way, and you can combine it with other vinegars that are less expensive. It comes as red or white. The red is the one I use the most.

Eggs — Eggs are a good source of protein, and I believe the jury is still out on how they affect cholesterol levels. However, the yolks contain a great deal of arachindonic acid, which can cause problems. I overdid the consumption of eggs last year, and I developed an angry rash across my upper chest and back. A little research revealed that the probable villain was arachindonic acid. I quit eating eggs immediately and the rash slowly cleared up.

Since then I have subtracted some of the yolks and added tofu to all of my egg dishes and have had no more trouble. You can also substitute egg replacers if you prefer.

Try to find yard eggs, as they are a more natural food and have a greater nutrient value than caged eggs.

Grapeseed Oil — My favorite oil other than olive oil. It is very mild and great for sautéing or using in dressings.

Herbamare — A delicious organic herbal seasoning salt. I use it often, but any herbal flavoring or salt substitute can be used in its place.

Kelp — A mild sea vegetable; in powdered form, it is used in addition to sea salt. Because most sea salt contains no iodine, kelp is a handy supplement. If you use a sea salt that contains iodine, omit the kelp.

Kombu — A sea vegetable that is normally used when cooking dried beans. It enhances their flavor, adds minerals and makes them more digestible. It is removed after cooking.

Kudzu (or sometimes Kuzu) — A white, wild-root starch used to thicken sauces, gravies and puddings. It is very alkalizing and soothing. It dissolves in cold water and thickens when cooked and is interchangeable with arrowroot.

Liquid Aminos — A soy bouillon developed by Paul Bragg. It is mineral rich, not as salty as soy sauce or tamari, and a great addition to some soups, sauces, gravies, dips, or what-have-you.

Sea salt — use instead of supermarket salt which contains additives and none of the minerals.

Sesame oil — An "oriental" oil with a unique flavor, good for stir-fries and oriental salads. The dark, or roasted kind is the most flavorful and should be added to stir-fry dishes after cooking. Try adding a small amount to a milder oil in oriental salads for an authentic taste.

Stevia — An herb sweetener. It comes in a white powder (found in the supplement section of a health food store) and is dissolved in water and measured in drops. Store in the refrigerator after dissolving. The powder will keep indefinitely unrefrigerated. Very, very sweet. Safe for diabetics.

Tahini — A sesame butter used as a replacement for butter or dairy in soups, sauces, dressings and dips.

Tamari — A wheat-free soy sauce, stronger in flavor than soy sauce.

Tekka — A rich, dark-brown seasoning made from greatly overcooked vegetables (my description). It adds a depth of flavor to gravy that I can't get any other way.

Tofu — Soybean curd that is a truly versatile, healthful, high-protein food. It comes in many varieties; the Japanese style called silken, is found in the little aseptic packages and the Chinese style, which is a firmer type, is packed in water in tubs.

Tofu, pressed — This is simply tofu that has had as much water as possible taken out. You can wrap it in dish towels or paper towels for an hour or so or set something heavy on it to "squeeze" out the water. Use the Chinese style, extra-firm tofu. It doesn't contain as much water to start with as the silken type.

Umeboshi — An oriental, salt-pickled plum with a sour/salty taste, usually used in salad dressings or cooked with vegetables. It is very alkalizing and good for upset stomachs. Umeboshi vinegar is a byproduct and I sometimes use it in place of vinegar or lemon juice (both acidic) when preparing a salad dressing accompanying a starchy (alkaline) meal. Be careful, however, it is very salty.

Vogue Vege Base — A vegetable powdered bouillon that turns water into an instant, delicious vegetable broth used in soups, sauces, dips and gravies. I couldn't cook without it. It does contain nutritional yeast, however, so if you have a yeast problem, you should make your own vegetable broth.

Most of the foods and seasonings I use that are not familiar to many Americans, I discovered when I studied macrobiotics. There are a great many books about macrobiotics and you might want to read one or two. (Some are listed in the back.) The natural health food movement owes a great deal to the leaders of macrobiotics, for they were quite instrumental in getting organic, whole foods into our marketplace.

Whatever you purchase, familiar or not, please start carefully reading the labels. So many items contain sugar in one form or another and a great number have preservatives, artificial color and other nonfood additives. No one should be ingesting these things, especially someone with health problems.

That applies to toothpaste, skin cream and deodorant also. Find items in health food stores or by mail order that contain only life enhancing substances. Your skin absorbs anything you put on it, so it is just as important to treat it well as it is to eat properly.

Chapter Thirty

◆

The Zen of Peeling, Chopping and Dicing

Since I am not that crazy about preparing food, the time it takes to prepare fresh fruits and vegetables was, at first, a source of irritation to me. I was accustomed to dumping canned or frozen foods in a pan and turning on the heat. In a short time, however, the new, sharp knives I acquired (my favorite is a light weight, broad-bladed Mac knife) and the time I spent learning to use them properly made the act a pleasant ritual, an actual time of meditation! Nothing else I do during the day is as quieting and peaceful as the repetitive and rhythmic motion of dicing a bunch of vegetables. Paying strict attention to the thing you are doing at the moment is "being here now."

I truly believe that we are the creators of our own reality. If we get up in the morning and it is raining, we have a choice to make about what kind of a day it is going to be for us. We have a tendency to put a label on it. "What a nasty day," we might say. The day, however, is just a day. A farmer down the road might be absolutely delighted that it is raining. If our own attitude toward this day, on which it happens to be raining, is one of peace or joy or pleasantness, we turn what could have been a "bad day" for us into a good one. Our minds do it, the universe doesn't "do it" to us.

So back to chopping vegetables. You can resent spending the time on something so mundane or you can turn it into a very pleasant experience. Your choice.

Have the chef at your favorite restaurant show you how to chop correctly if you don't already know. The tip of the knife stays on the cutting board and your arm resembles the connector between the wheels on a train. It is smooth and rhythmic and quieting to the mind.

Chapter Thirty-one

◆

Two Useful Lists

To assist you in discovering the foods to which you might be sensitive, I have listed below the ones that are common troublemakers.

baking yeast	peanuts	cow products
crab	pork	wheat
tomatoes	mushrooms	shellfish
brewer's yeast	oranges	grapefruit
lemon	peppers	walnuts
beef	eggplant	honey

That should give you a start. There are a number of books about food allergies in the book stores.

Some alternative practitioners believe that applied kinesiology is a valid means of determining food sensitivities.

Applied kinesiology is an offshoot of chiropractic medicine. People who believe in it maintain that muscle function reflects physical health. To evaluate your sensitivity to a food, a practitioner will have you hold one arm out, shoulder high with your palm facing down. The practitioner will then push down on your arm to test your muscle strength. The resistance encountered is your "norm." You then put a suspected food in your mouth and your arm is pushed down again. If you are sensitive to that particular food, these applied Kinesiologists maintain that your arm strength is weaker. I have tried this test on a number of people using white sugar. In each case, my test subjects and I were incredulous at the weakness of their muscles with sugar in their mouths. I can't tell if this works with foods other than sugar. The results were much less decisive when we tested other foods.

Some testers have you hold the tips of your index finger and thumb together while you hold a substance in the other hand. Then they try to pull your thumb and finger apart. Having been tested a number of times both ways, I have to say that my muscle strength did seem to vary considerably and did respond the same way again and again to the same substances. I am inclined to recommend it and you might want to pursue it further.

Dr. Rosenfeld, in his *Guide to Alternative Medicine*, says he doesn't believe in applied kinesiology. He tested several of his patients with known food allergies and couldn't sense any difference in their muscle strength.

It is possible that those who use it are more sensitive to the difference in muscle strength than Dr. Rosenfeld, simply because they have practiced applied kinesiology for some time. Perhaps not. We have to trust our own judgement. There are several books on the subject if you are interested.

The good news is that, once your immune system and digestive system have calmed down, you are much less apt to react to so many substances. I can even tolerate lemon juice now, as long as I don't try it too often.

Dividing Foods Into Three Categories:

ACID
(Proteins and acid fruits)

Protein
all soy products
all nuts and peanuts
meat (beef, pork, chicken, turkey, etc.)
fish and seafood
eggs
milk and dairy

Fruit
lime
lemon
grapefruit
tomato (cooked)
cranberries
rhubarb
apple cider vinegar

NEUTRAL
(Fats, oils and vegetables)

Fats and oils

(The following are the suggested oils only)
butter (sparingly)
canola oil
grapeseed oil
olive oil
sesame oil and seeds
sunflower and pumpkin seeds

Neutral vegetables

asparagus	garlic	peppers
avocado	green beans	radishes
beets	greens	rutabaga
broccoli	kale	spinach
Brussel sprouts	kohlrabi	sprouts
cabbage	leek	tomato (raw)
carrots	lettuce	turnip
celery	mushrooms	watercress
cucumber	okra	wax beans
eggplant	onion	zucchini
endive	parsley	
escarole	peas	

ALKALINE
(Starchy vegetables, grains, fruit and sweeteners)

all grains and	potato (sweet)	all sweeteners
flour products	potato (white)	such as:
beans (dry)	pumpkin	honey
carob	winter squash	maple syrup
corn	all fruit not	grain syrups
peas (dry)	listed under acid	Exception:
parsnips		stevia

(Artichokes are neutral, but Jerusalem artichokes are a starchy vegetable.)

Please, *always* keep in mind that fresh, raw vegetables that still contain living enzymes are important in our diet. On a daily basis you should consume at least 70% of your vegetables raw. That means less cooking and more free time! Lean on the salad recipes for a great part of your daily intake, or serve a tray of raw vegetables with a dip or two before meals.

Recipes

Acid-Protein

Appetizers

Garlic-Ripe Olive Dip 124
Warm Artichoke Dip 125
Little Protein Dippers 126
Tofu-Onion Dip 127
Guacamole-Tofu Dip 128
Quick Guacamole 128

Soups

Broccoli-Soy Cheese Soup 129
Cream of Tomato Soup 130
Gazpacho 130
Zucchini Bisque 131
Vegetable Soup 132
Shrimp Bisque 133
Cream of Asparagus Soup 134
Manhattan Fish Chowder 135
Cream of Mushroom Soup 136

Salads

Caesar Crab Salad 137
Caesar Salad 138

Green Salad & Pecans with Ginger Dressing 139
Spinach Salad with Dijon Dressing 140
Vegetable Salad with Creamy Ranch Dressing 141
Grilled Vegetable Salad 142
Salmon Salad 143
Tuna Salad in Stuffed Tomato 143
Shrimp Louis 144
Mushroom-Tomato Salad 145
Oriental Salad 146
Green Goddess Dressing 147

Tofu Dishes

Oriental Broccoli Quiche Sans Crust 148
Asparagus Quiche Sans Crust 149
Spinach Quiche Sans Crust 150
Broccoli-Tofu Souffle 151
Blackened Tofu 152
Tofu Squares 152
Indonesian Tofu 153
Lemon Tofu Nuggets 153
Tofu-Mushroom Pancake 155
Creamy Veggie Bake 156
Curried Tofu 157
Grilled Tofu Steaks 158
Tofu Loaf 158
Tofu-Cauliflower Casserole 160
Szechuan Tofu and Stir Fried Vegetables 161

Egg Dishes

Basic Omelet 162
Omelet Variations 163
Spanish Omelet Sauce 164
Vegetable Omelet 165
Scrambled Eggs 166
Deviled Eggs 166
Zucchini Pancake 167

Recipes

Seafood

Fish Dijon 168
Fish Fromage 169
Fish with Artichokes 170
Baked Fish with Horseradish-Mayonnaise 170
Broiled Fish with Almond Pesto 171
Grilled Tuna with Teriyaki Sauce 172
Shrimp Creole 173
Crab and Mushroom Bake 174
Deviled Crab 175
Barbecued Salmon 176
Shrimp-Cashew Szechuan Stir Fry 177
Tuna Casserole 178
Salmon Patties with Mustard Sauce 179
Poached Fish with Mushrooms 180
Canned Tuna Bake 181

Vegetables

Savory Brussels Sprouts 182
Zucchini with Ginger and Cashews 183
Mushroom-Zucchini Puff 184
Zucchini with Fresh Basil 185
Puréed Eggplant 185
Broccoli-Red Bell Pepper Stir Fry 186
Green Beans Almondine 187
Cauliflower with Peanut Sauce 188
Broccoli Casserole 189
Stuffed Zucchini 190

Sauces and Gravies

Cashew Sauce 191
Almond Ginger Sauce 191
Jalapeño-Dill Sauce 192
Peanut Sauce 192
Lemon Sauce 193

Soy Cheese Sauce 193
Cashew-Ginger Sauce 194
Sweet and Sour Sauce 194
Barbeque Sauce 195
Roasted Pecan Gravy 195

Desserts

Butterscotch Mousse 196
Lemon Mousse 197
Mocha Mousse with Toasted Pecans 198

Neutral

Appetizers

Vegetable Plate 199
Roasted Red Pepper Dip 199

Soups

Neutral Gazpacho 200
Vegetable Soup 201
Quick Steamed Vegetable Soup 202
Cool Avocado Soup 202
Puréed Carrot Soup 203

Salads

Great American Green Salad 204
Oriental Salad 205
Crunchy Mexican Salad 206
Southwest Slaw 207

Vegetables

Steamed Vegetables 208
Dilled Baby Beets 209

Four Color Stir-Fry 209
Stir Fried Kale with Garlic 210
Balsamic Glazed Onions 210
Puréed Vegetables with Roasted Garlic 211
Carrots with Coriander 212
Roasted Vegetables 213
Garlic Green Beans or Broccoli 214
Baked Carrots and Onions 214
Carrots, Zucchini and Peas 215
Steamed Cabbage 215

Sauces

Red Bell Pepper Sauce 216
Mushroom Sauce 216
Quick Brown Sauce 217
White Wine Sauce 217
Shiitaki Gravy 218

Alkaline-Starch

Appetizers

Lentil Paté 219
Aduki Bean Dip 220
Carrot Paté 221
White Bean Paté 222
Red Bell Pepper Dip 222
Mushroom Crostini 223
Roasted Garbanzo Beans 223
Roasted Sweet Onion-Garlic Spread 224
Baked Garlic 224

Soups

Baked Potato Soup 225
Lima Bean Soup 226
Lentil Soup 227

Healing Vegetable Soup 228
Split Pea Soup 229
Golden Bisque 230
Quick Black Bean Soup 230
Quick Cream of Celery Soup 231

Sandwich Suggestions

Salads

Complete Meal Quinoa Salad 232
Quinoa-Stir Fry Vegetable Salad 233
Garbanzo Salad 234
Black-eyed Pea & Sweet Potato Salad 234
Southwest Lentil Salad 235
Texas Caviar 236
Taco Salad 237
Spanish Rice Salad 238
White Bean-Horseradish Salad 239
Chinese Quinoa Salad 240

Vegetables

Butternut Squash-Orange Purée 242
Pineapple-Glazed Carrots 242
Braised Red Cabbage 243
Sweet Fall Squash Medley 244
Acorn Squash Purée 245
Baked Garlic Potatoes 246
Scalloped Potatoes 237
Stuffed Squash 248
Spiced Mixed "Fries" 249
Sherried Sweet Potatoes 249

Sauces

Brown Mushroom Sauce 250
Stir Fry Sauce 251

Beautiful Beet Sauce 251
Orange-Ginger Sauce 252
Sweet and Sour Sauce 252

Breads

Chapati 253
Garbanzo Chapati 254
Rye Flatbreads 254
Corn Bread 255
Sesame Bread Sticks 256
Mexican Corn Bread 256
Corn Crisps 257
Whole Wheat Biscuits 257
Oatmeal Crackers 258
Lemon-Poppyseed Muffins 259
Apricot-Millet Muffins 260

Desserts

Baked Apple 261
Pineapple-Ginger Sorbet 262
Oat Pie Crust 262
Vanilla Pudding 263
Peach Cream Pie 263
Strawberry or Blueberry Cream Pie 264
"Apple Pie" Filling 265
Crepes 266
Cherry Sauce 267
Pear Crisp 267
Plain Cake 268
Raspberry Sauce 269
Strawberry Sauce 269
Fresh Blueberry Sauce 270

ACID-PROTEIN

APPETIZERS

Garlic-Ripe Olive Dip

1 1/2 teaspoons minced garlic
1/3 cup raw cashew pieces
1 package silken, firm tofu
2 tablespoons fresh lemon juice
1/4 teaspoon sea salt
dash cayenne
2 tablespoons capers, drained
1/4 cup pitted Kalamata olives

1. In a processor, cream garlic and cashew pieces, adding tofu and lemon juice a little at a time.
2. Add sea salt, cayenne, and capers and process until smooth and creamy.
3. Add olives and process just until the olives are cut into bits. Transfer to a bowl and stir to mix well. Refrigerate, covered until ready to serve.

Serve with little protein dippers or fresh, raw vegetables. Some suggestions: cucumber sticks, jicama, celery sticks, red pepper, and zucchini or yellow squash.

Warm Artichoke Dip

1/4 cup raw cashew pieces
1/3 cup pure water
2 tablespoons fresh lemon juice
1/3 cup light mayonnaise
1 teaspoon Dijon mustard
1 teaspoon arrowroot
1 teaspoon minced garlic
1/4 cup grated soy Parmesan
1 14-ounce can artichoke hearts, drained

1. Heat oven to 375 degrees.
2. In a processor, purée cashews in water and lemon juice until smooth.
3. Add mayonnaise, mustard, arrowroot, garlic and soy Parmesan and process again until thoroughly mixed.
4. Add artichoke hearts and process just until artichoke is finely chopped.
5. Oil a one-quart casserole and spoon mixture into it. Bake about 20 minutes, until bubbly.

Serve with little protein dippers, endive leaves, raw turnip slices, jicama, or zucchini rounds.

Little Protein Dippers

1 egg
3 egg whites
1/2 cup soy powder
1/2 cup water
1/4 teaspoon sea salt

1. Combine ingredients in a blender and blend until smooth.
2. Wipe a skillet with oil and heat until a drop of water sizzles and skips.
3. Drop batter by tablespoons in skillet and cook until dry on top, turn and cook until lightly brown on the other side.

These are like minature pancakes that can be used in a variety of ways. They will substitute for crackers (although they are soft) to use with the dips, or made larger and used for crepes, pancakes, or in place of pasta. Add garlic powder to the basic recipe for Italian dishes or try onion powder and dill for an all protein "bread" for open faced "sandwiches."

Tofu-Onion Dip

1/3 cup water
1/3 cup raw cashew pieces
1/2 package silken firm tofu, light
2 teaspoons cider vinegar
1/2 teaspoon powdered garlic
2 tablespoons fresh, minced parsley
1/2 teaspoon tamari
2 tablespoons instant minced onion
Herbamare and cayenne to taste

1. In a processor, purée cashews in the water until smooth.
2. Add the tofu, vinegar, garlic, parsley, and tamari and process again until smooth.
3. Add the minced onion and process until just mixed.
4. Transfer to a bowl and stir in Herbamare and cayenne to taste.
5. Refrigerate about an hour to let flavors develop.

Good with all kinds of fresh, raw, or lightly steamed vegetables. (Always steam broccoli for about three minutes. It is much easier to digest.)

Guacamole-Tofu Dip

2 ripe Haas avocados
2 teaspoons minced garlic
2 tablespoons white balsamic vinegar
1 tablespoon fresh lemon juice
2 teaspoons Herbamare
1/2 package silken tofu, firm, light
1 large, ripe organic tomato, diced
1/3 cup minced sweet onion

1. In a processor, combine all but the tomato and onion. Purée until smooth.
2. Transfer to a bowl and stir in the tomato and onion. Serve immediately or chill, covered, for a few hours.

This dip is good with celery or jicama sticks, any other fresh, raw vegetable or little protein dippers.

Quick Guacamole

2 large ripe Haas avocados
1 tablespoon fresh lemon juice
4 tablespoons Pace's Chunky Picante Sauce (mild, medium, or hot depending on your taste)

1. Mash the avocados with a fork. Add lemon juice and picante sauce and mix well. Serve immediately or cover surface with plastic wrap and refrigerate until ready to serve.
2. Serve guacamole on a bed of lettuce.

Serves 4.

PROTEIN - ACID SOUPS

Broccoli-Soy Cheese Soup

1 tablespoon olive oil
1 small onion, chopped
4 peeled stems of broccoli, chopped
2 cups water
1 tablespoon Vogue Vege Broth
1 teaspoon sea salt
1/4 teaspoon kelp
1/8 teaspoon cayenne
1 teaspoon Herbamare seasoning
1/2 cup raw cashew pieces blended in 1 cup water
2 cups grated Soya Kaas cheddar-style cheese
4 cups of quite small broccoli florets, steamed for 3 minutes, plunged
     in cold water, drained, then set aside

1. In a soup pot, sauté onion in the oil for 5 minutes.
2. Stir in Vege Base, water, broccoli stems and seasonings. Bring to a boil and simmer for 20 minutes.
3 Add half of the steamed broccoli florets to the stems mixture and purée in batches in the blender and return to the soup pot.
4. Add cashew cream and the soy cheese. Heat, stirring frequently until the cheese melts.
5. Add the other half of the broccoli florets and stir for a few seconds, until the broccoli is heated through.

Serves 4.

Cream of Tomato Soup

1 14.5-ounce can diced organic tomatoes
3 cups almond milk
1/2 teaspoon tarragon
1 teaspoon Herbamare
1 1/2 tablespoons arrowroot dissolved in 1/4 cup water

1. Purée tomatoes, almond milk, tarragon, and Herbamare in a blender. Pour mixture in a large saucepan and bring to a boil.
2. Turn heat down to medium-low and stir in arrowroot mixture. Simmer, stirring constantly until thickened.

Serves 4.

Gazpacho

2 11.5-ounce cans tomato juice
1 14.5-ounce can organic, diced tomatoes
3 medium cucumbers, peeled, seeded and chopped
1 green bell pepper, seeded and chopped
1 red bell pepper, seeded and chopped
1/2 medium onion, chopped
1/3 cup minced parsley
1/2 teaspoon garlic powder
2 tablespoons balsamic vinegar
1 teaspoon sea salt
1 tablespoon Spike seasoning (or other no-salt seasoning)
1 teaspoon Worcestershire sauce
Few drops Tobasco sauce

1. Combine all ingredients in a blender and blend briefly, until well mixed but not smooth. Adjust seasonings.
2. Chill for several hours to allow flavors to blend.

Serves 4.

Zucchini Bisque

1 tablespoon olive oil
2 onions, chopped
2 carrots, finely chopped
4 medium zucchini, chopped
1 tablespoon sea salt
1 cup white wine
3 tablespoons Vogue Vege Base
Dash of kelp and cayenne
1 tablespoon fresh lemon juice
1 10 1/2-ounce package silken, firm tofu
4 cups water
1/4 cup minced fresh parsley

1. In a soup pot, sauté vegetables in oil and salt for 10 minutes.
2. Meanwhile, in a blender, cream the wine, Vege base, kelp, cayenne, lemon juice, tofu and water until smooth.
3. Add the wine-tofu mixture to the vegetables in the soup pot. Bring to a boil and simmer another 5 minutes.
4 Purée soup in batches in a blender until smooth. Return to heat for 2 more minutes. Serve garnished with minced parsley.

Serves 4.

Vegetable Soup

1 tablespoon olive oil
1 medium onion, minced
2 large carrots, cut in thin rounds
2 stalks celery, chopped
1 tablespoon Vogue Vege Base
5 cups water
2 cups trimmed, chopped green beans
1/4 head, small green cabbage, shredded
1 14.5-ounce can organic, diced tomatoes
1 medium zucchini, cut into rounds
4 small yellow crook-neck squash, cut into rounds
1 teaspoon Herbamare
1 1/2 tablespoons apple cider vinegar
Salt and cayenne to taste

1. In a large soup pot, sauté onion, carrot and celery in oil for 5 minutes.
2. Stir in Vege Base
3. Add water, green beans, cabbage and tomatoes and bring to a boil.
4. Reduce heat, cover and simmer for 30 minutes.
5. Add the remaining ingredients and simmer another 10 minutes.

Serves 4.

Shrimp Bisque

1 tablespoon olive oil
1/2 medium onion, diced
1 stalk celery, diced
1/2 pound medium-size shrimp, peeled, deveined, and chopped
I bay leaf
1 teaspoon dried thyme
1 cup white wine
1 tablespoon Vogue Vege Base
1/2 teaspoon Herbamare
1/8 teaspoon cayenne
1 14.5-ounce can organic, diced tomatoes
3 cups water
1/2 cup raw cashew pieces
1/4 cup minced parsley

1. In a soup pot, sauté onion, and celery in the oil for 5 minutes.
2. Add bay leaf, thyme, wine, Vege Base, Herbamare, cayenne, tomatoes and 3 cups of the water and simmer for 30 minutes.
3. Add shrimp and cook 3 minutes.
4. In the meantime, blend the cashew pieces in the remaining cup of water until very smooth.
5. Remove bay leaf from shrimp mixture and, in batches, blend the mixture with the cashew cream, leaving small bits of shrimp intact.
6. Pour blended mixture back into the soup pot, stir to mix, and reheat.
7. Garnish with minced parsley.

Serves 4.

Cream of Asparagus Soup

2 1/2 cups water
1 cup white wine
1 pound fresh asparagus
1/2 onion, chopped
1 stalk celery, chopped
1/2 teaspoon minced garlic
1 tablespoon fresh lemon juice
1 10.5-ounce package silken, firm tofu, crumbled
1/2 teaspoon sea salt
1/4 teaspoon ground coriander
1/8 cup minced parsley

1. Remove 1-inch tips from asparagus and, in a large sauce pan, boil in the water for 2 minutes. Remove tips and set aside. Chop when cool.
2. Peel tough stems and chop the rest of the asparagus.
3. Add wine, onion, asparagus stems, celery and garlic to the water. Bring to a boil. Simmer, covered, for 30 minutes.
4. In two batches, blend the cooked asparagus mixture until smooth. In the second batch, add the crumbled tofu, lemon juice and seasonings, and blend just until completely mixed.
5. Return blended mixtures to the saucepan, stir well to mix, add the chopped asparagus tips, and reheat.
6. Garnish with minced parsley.

Serves 4.

Manhattan Fish Chowder

3/4 pound firm, white fish fillets
1/2 lemon, thinly sliced
3 cups water
1/2 cup white wine
1 tablespoon oil
1 medium onion, diced
1 stalk celery, diced
1/2 green pepper, diced
1 small carrot, diced
1/2 head cauliflower florets
1 14.5-ounce can organic, diced tomatoes*
1 cup almond cream (see below)
1/4 cup finely sliced scallions

1. Place fish, lemon, water and wine in a saucepan. Bring to a boil, reduce heat, cover and simmer for about 12 minutes, just until fish flakes easily with a fork.
2 Remove fish and lemon slices from stock and let cool slightly. When cool enough to handle, chop fish into bite size pieces and set aside.
3. In a soup pot, sauté onion, celery, pepper, and carrot for 10 minutes.
4. Add soup stock, tomatoes, and cauliflower, bring to a boil and simmer, covered, for 20 minutes.
5. Stir in almond cream and bring just to a simmer.
6. Add fish to soup and heat 1 minute.
7. Garnish with scallions.

Serves 4.

(To make almond cream, blend 3/4 cup of blanched almonds in 1 cup of water until smooth. Strain by pouring through a fine sieve).
*If you are sensitive to cooked tomatoes leave them out and add 3/4 cup of water. Then you have a regular fish chowder.

Cream of Mushroom Soup

1 tablespoon oil
1/2 pound mushrooms, chopped (button mushrooms or a mixture of
    button and exotic mushrooms)
1/2 onion, chopped
1 teaspoon minced garlic
1/3 cup dry sherry
1 tablespoon Vogue Vege Base
4 cups water, divided
1/3 cup raw cashew pieces
sea salt and cayenne pepper to taste

1. In a large saucepan, sauté mushrooms and onions in oil
   for 10 minutes.
2. Add garlic, sherry, Vege Base, and 3 cups of water.
   Cover and simmer for 15 minutes.
3. In the meantime, blend the cashew pieces in the
   remaining cup of water.
4. In batches, blend the mushroom mixture and the
   cashew mixture together, leaving small pieces of
   mushroom intact.
5 Return everything to the pot and bring to a simmer.
   Season to taste with salt and cayenne.

Serves 4.

ACID - PROTEIN SALADS

Caesar Crab Salad

1/4 cup light mayonnaise
1 teaspoon white balsamic vinegar
1 teaspoon Dijon mustard
2 teaspoons Worcestershire sauce
1 teaspoon fresh lemon juice
2 sprigs parsley, minced
2 green onions, finely sliced
1/3 cup red cabbage, shredded
1 stalk celery, diced
1 tomato, diced
2 teaspoons capers, drained
2 6-ounce cans lump crabmeat, rinsed and drained
Head of Romaine lettuce

1. Combine first 5 ingredients and mix well.
2. Add the rest of the ingredients, except the lettuce, and stir together.
3. Serve on a large bed of torn lettuce leaves.

Serves 4.

Caesar Salad

Dressing:
1 oil-packed dried tomato, well drained
3 kalamata or other black olives, pitted
1 teaspoon Dijon mustard
1/8 cup raw cashew pieces
1 tablespoon olive oil*
1 tablespoon fresh lemon juice
1 teaspoon balsamic vinegar
1/2 teaspoon minced garlic
2 teaspoons Worcestershire sauce
Sea salt to taste
Large head of romaine lettuce

Optional: Sprinkle with soy Parmesan

1. Put all the dressing ingredients in a processor and process until smooth.
2. Wash, dry, and tear romaine leaves and put in a large salad bowl.
3. Just before serving, toss with dressing and transfer to salad plates.

Serves 2.

*Always use extra-virgin olive oil

Green Salad And Pecans
With Ginger Dressing

Mixed salad greens for 4
1/3 cup chopped pecans

Dressing:
1 teaspoon grated fresh ginger
3/4 of a package of silken tofu, firm
1/4 cup water
1 teaspoon sea salt
2 tablespoons sesame oil
3 tablespoons brown rice vinegar

1. Combine dressing ingredients in a processor and process until smooth.
2. Wash, dry, and tear salad greens and divide equally on 4 salad plates.
3. Drizzle greens with dressing and sprinkle pecans over the salads.

Spinach Salad With Dijon Dressing

2 bunches of fresh spinach
1 large Haas avocado
1/4 large sweet onion

Dressing:
2 tablespoons Dijon mustard
1/4 cup olive oil
1/8 cup balsamic vinegar
1/8 cup apple cider vinegar
1/2 teaspoon sea salt
dash of cayenne

1. Separate leaves of spinach and immerse in a large basin of water. Agitate spinach to release sand. Lift spinach from water and drain, washing away sand. Fill basin with fresh water and repeat process to clean the spinach thoroughly. Remove stems and dry leaves with towels. Arrange on 4 plates.
2. Peel avocado, remove pit, and slice into 8 sections. Put 2 sections on each plate.
3. Peel and slice onion. Separate into rings and arrange rings equally on the plates.
4. Whisk together the dressing ingredients and drizzle equally on the salads.

Serves 4.

Vegetable Salad With Creamy Ranch Dressing

Use your favorite raw vegetables on top of a bed of lettuce.

Dressing:
2 green onions, white and green parts, chopped
1 teaspoon minced garlic
1 tablespoon white balsamic vinegar
1 tablespoon lemon juice
1 10.5-ounce package silken tofu, firm
1 teaspoon oregano
1 tablespoon grapeseed oil
salt to taste
few drops of stevia to taste
water as needed

1. In a processor, purée all dressing ingredients until very smooth. Add and process small amounts of pure water if dressing is too thick. Let sit 15 or 20 minutes. Will keep in the refrigerator up to three days.
2. Arrange vegetables on salad plates and pile a large spoonful of dressing in the center.

Serves up to 8.

Grilled Vegetable Salad

Marinade:
1/3 cup balsamic vinegar
1/8 cup olive oil
2 teaspoons minced garlic
1 teaspoon Italian seasoning
1/4 teaspoon sea salt
drops of stevia to taste

4 carrots
2 sweet red peppers
2 zucchini
2 yellow squash
1 large sweet onion
1 cup soy mozzarella cut in cubes

1. Combine marinade ingredients in a large bowl. Set aside.
2. Cut vegetables into large pieces and stir into marinade. Soak at least 30 minutes, stirring occasionally.
3. Drain vegetables, reserving marinade.
4. Cook vegetables in a grill basket over hot coals for 15 to 20 minutes.
5. Return vegetables to marinade and toss gently. Refrigerate several hours or overnight, covered.
6. Mix in soy mozzarella cubes and serve on a bed of leaf lettuce.

Serves 4.

Salmon Salad

2 6 1/2-ounce cans red salmon, skin and bones removed and well
    drained
1/3 cup light mayonnaise
1 stalk celery, minced
1/8 cup minced red onion
2 tablespoons minced fresh dill
1 tablespoon fresh lemon juice
2 or 3 dashes cayenne

1. Crumble salmon and combine with all the other ingredients.
2. Serve on a bed of lettuce garnished with cherry tomato halves, celery sticks, and a lemon wedge.

Serves 4.

Tuna Salad In Stuffed Tomato

1 6-ounce can solid white tuna packed in water
2 stalks celery, diced
1/2 cup sweet onion, diced
1/4 cup minced dill pickle
1/3 cup toasted almonds, chopped
1/3 cup light mayonnaise
2 ripe, organic tomatoes
Leaf lettuce
Kalamata olives

1. Drain and flake tuna.
2. Stir tuna together with the rest of the ingredients.
3. Core tomatoes and cut into 6 sections from the top almost through the bottom. Place on lettuce leaves.
4. Pile tuna salad on top of tomatoes.
5. Garnish with olives.

Serves 2.

Shrimp Louis Salad

2 pounds cooked, peeled, cold shrimp
1 cup light mayonnaise
1/2 cup tomato sauce
1 tablespoon Worcestershire sauce
2 teaspoons prepared horseradish
1/4 cup minced dill pickle
1 stalk celery, minced
1 green onion, thinly sliced
2 tablespoons minced parsley
1/4 teaspoon cayenne

1. Mix together all ingredients except the shrimp.
2. Add the shrimp and stir lightly to coat shrimp with the dressing.
3. Arrange shrimp on beds of lettuce and sprinkle with paprika.
4. Garnish with celery sticks, radishes, cherry tomatoes, and/or lemon wedges.

Serves 4.

Mushroom-Tomato Salad

1 teaspoon olive oil
1/4 cup dry sherry
1/2 cup diced onions
2 cups mushrooms (your choice) thinly sliced
2 tablespoons lemon juice
1 teaspoon chives or green onion, minced
2 organic tomatoes, sliced
leaf lettuce leaves

1. Combine oil, sherry, onions, and mushrooms in a large skillet. Sauté over medium heat for about 15 minutes, stirring frequently.
2. Remove from heat and stir in lemon juice and chives (or green onions).
3. Arrange lettuce on salad plates and place sliced tomatoes on the lettuce.
4. Spoon warm mushroom mixture on top of tomatoes.

Serves 2.

Oriental Salad

Dressing:
1 package silken, firm tofu
3 tablespoons scallions (white part)
2 teaspoons minced garlic
1 tablespoon freshly grated ginger
1/8 teaspoon cayenne
1/4 cup rice wine vinegar
3 tablespoons tamari
2 teaspoons dark sesame oil
few drops of stevia, to taste
water to thin

Combine all ingredients in a processor or blender and process until smooth, adding water to desired thickness.

Salad:
Make a slaw using your favorite kind of cabbage, slivers of red bell pepper, and julienned snow peas. (Or any other favorite or on-hand raw vegetables.)
Place vegetables on salad plates and spoon on the dressing. (Any extra dressing will keep for several days in a closed container in the refrigerator.)

This makes enough dressing for 8 salads.

Green Goddess Dressing

1 package silken, firm tofu
2 tablespoons flat leaf parsley, chopped
2 tablespoons fresh basil, chopped
2 tablespoons scallion greens, chopped
1 tablespoon capers
2 teaspoons minced garlic
3 tablespoons white balsamic vinegar
3 tablespoons extra virgin olive oil
several drops of stevia, to taste
1/2 teaspoon salt
water to thin

Combine all ingredients in a processor or blender and processes until smooth, using water to get desired thickness.

Use this dressing on any raw salad or plain salad greens. It will keep for several days in a covered container in the refrigerator.

Tofu

Oriental Broccoli Quiche Sans Crust

3 1/2 cups broccoli florets and peeled, finely chopped stems,
steamed 3 minutes
2 packages silken tofu, extra-firm
2 tablespoons water
3 tablespoons tahini
1 1/2 tablespoons umeboshi paste
1 tablespoon tamari
1/3 cup minced roasted red pepper
1/3 cup minced green onion

1. Heat oven to 400 degrees.
2. In a food processor, combine tofu, water, tahini, umeboshi paste and tamari. Process until smooth and creamy.
3. In a bowl, combine broccoli, red pepper and green onion. Pour tofu mixture into the vegetables and mix well.
4. Pour the mixture into an oiled pie dish bake for 25 to 30 minutes. (Until a knife inserted in the middle comes out clean.)
5. Let sit for 15 minutes before serving.

Serves 4.

Asparagus Quiche Sans Crust

1 tablespoon olive oil
1 1/2 cup minced onion
2 cups asparagus, (peel tough stalks) cut in half-inch pieces
2 tablespoons water
2 packages silken tofu, extra-firm
1 1/2 tablespoons cider vinegar
2 tablespoons Dijon mustard
3 tablespoons tahini
1/2 teaspoon marjoram
1/2 teaspoon basil
1/2 cup minced fresh parsley

1. Heat oven to 400 degrees. Oil pie dish.
2. Sauté onion in oil for 5 minutes.
3. Add green onions, asparagus and water. Put on lid and steam about 4 minutes Remove lid and remove from heat.
4. In a processor, combine tofu and the rest of the ingredients except the parsley. Process until smooth and creamy.
5. Add parsley and process just until well mixed.
6. Spoon any remaining water out of the skillet and stir tofu mixture into the vegetables.
7. Spoon mixture into the pie dish and bake for 25 to 30 minutes. (Until a knife comes out clean).
8. Let sit for 15 minutes before serving.

Serves 4.

Spinach Quiche Sans Crust

1 tablespoon olive oil
1 3/4 cup minced onion
2 teaspoons minced garlic
2 cups fresh spinach, stems removed and chopped, or 1 10-ounce
    package of frozen spinach, thawed and drained
3/4 teaspoon nutmeg
2 packages silken tofu, extra-firm
1 1/2 tablespoons apple cider vinegar
3 tablespoons tahini
2 tablespoons Dijon mustard
1/2 teaspoon salt

1. Heat oven to 400 degrees, oil pie dish
2. Sauté onion in oil until translucent
3. Add garlic, spinach and nutmeg and sauté one more minute. Remove from heat
4. In a food processor, combine tofu, vinegar, tahini, mustard and salt. Process until smooth and creamy.
5. Add tofu mixture to the spinach and stir to mix well.
6. Spoon into pie dish and bake for 25 to 30 minutes. (Until a knife comes out clean).
7. Let sit for 15 minutes before serving.

Serves 4.

Broccoli-Tofu Souffle

4 cups broccoli, stems peeled and chopped, florets cut in small pieces.
1 10.5-ounce package silken, firm tofu
2 tablespoons lemon juice
1 teaspoon Herbamare
1 teaspoon fines herbs
1 1/2 cups grated cheddar soy cheese
1 1/2 tablespoon grapeseed oil
1 tablespoon Vogue Vege Base
1/3 cup water
1/2 cup soy milk or almond milk
1 1/4 teaspoons baking powder

1. Heat oven to 325 degrees.
2. Steam broccoli for 4 minutes.
3. In a processor, cream tofu. Add broccoli, lemon juice, Herbamare, and fines herbs and process until thoroughly blended.
4. Transfer to a large bowl.
5. In the processor, combine oil, Vege Base, cheese, water, and milk.
6. Stir Vege Base mixture into tofu mixture.
7. Spray an oven-proof casserole.
8. Stir the baking powder into the tofu mixture.
9. Pour into the casserole and bake for 45 minutes. Serve immediately.

Serves 4 to 6.

Blackened Tofu

1 tub of Chinese-style, extra-firm tofu, pressed
2 tablespoons lemon juice
2 tablespoons liquid aminos
2 tablespoons Cajun spice blend

1. Cut tofu in 1/2" thick slices.
2. Combine lemon juice and liquid aminos and marinate the tofu for 30 minutes.
3. Put spice blend in a plastic bag and add tofu, shaking to coat the tofu evenly.
4. Cook on outside grill for about 8 minutes on each side.

Serves 6.

Tofu Squares

1/2 package Chinese-style firm tofu, pressed
1/4 cup tamari
1 teaspoon grated fresh ginger
3 tablespoons balsamic vinegar
1/4 teaspoon dry mustard
1 tablespoon minced garlic
2 tablespoons grape seed oil

1. Cut tofu into thin slices.
2. Combine all the other ingredients except the oil.
3. Marinate the tofu for at least 1 hour, preferably several, in the refrigerator, turning once or twice.
4. Heat oil in a large skillet and sauté tofu until it is brown on both sides.
5. Heat the remaining marinade and serve with the tofu.

Serves 2 to 3.

Indonesian Tofu

1/2 package of Chinese-style, extra-firm tofu, pressed
2 teaspoons sesame oil
1 1/2 teaspoons minced garlic
2 teaspoons grated fresh ginger
Few dashes cayenne
3/4 cup water
1 teaspoon Vege Base
1/4 cup natural peanut butter
1 tablespoon tamari
1 tablespoon lemon juice
1 teaspoon apple cider vinegar
1/4 teaspoon salt

1. Heat oven to 350 degrees.
2. Spray a heat-proof dish with oil.
3. Heat the oil in a saucepan and sauté the garlic for 2 minutes.
4. Add the ginger and cayenne and sauté for 2 more minutes.
5. Stir in the Vege Base, then the water and simmer, covered, for 10 minutes.
6. Whisk in the peanut butter and tamari and cook, stirring, until the sauce thickens.
7. Whisk in the lemon juice, vinegar, and salt and cook 3 minutes longer.
8. Cut tofu into thin slices and arrange on the dish.
9. Pour the sauce evenly over the tofu and bake for 30 minutes.

Garnish with minced scallions if desired.

Serves 4 .

Lemon-Tofu Nuggets

1 tub of Chinese-style extra-firm tofu, pressed
1/2 cup fresh lemon juice
2 tablespoons balsamic vinegar
1/4 cup tamari
2 tablespoons minced fresh rosemary or 2 teaspoons dried
1/2 teaspoon sea salt
1/4 teaspoon kelp
1/8 teaspoon cayenne

1. Heat oven the 350 degrees.
2. Cut tofu in to 1/2 inch cubes and spread out on a glass baking dish.
3. Combine all the other ingredients, whisk together, and pour over tofu.
4. Bake for about 45 minutes, until the tofu has absorbed most of the marinade.
5. Cool in the marinade.

This will keep for about 3 days in the refrigerator in a tightly covered dish. It can be served with vegetables or in a salad.

Serves 6 to 8.

Tofu-Mushroom Pancake

1 package silken, firm tofu
2 tablespoons liquid aminos
1 tablespoon grapeseed oil
1 teaspoon Herbamare
1/2 medium-sized onion, diced
2 cups sliced mushrooms
1/2 green pepper, diced
1/2 red pepper, diced
1 carrot, scrubbed and diced
1 tablespoon grapeseed oil
2 scallions, minced, for garnish

1. Combine tofu, aminos, 1 tablespoon oil, and Herbamare in a processor until smooth.
2. Sauté all the vegetables and mushrooms in the other tablespoon oil in a large skillet until soft. (About 10 minutes.)
3. Spread the vegetables evenly in the skillet and gently pour the tofu mixture over the vegetables.
4. Cook until golden brown, turning once. Garnish with minced scallions.

Serves 4.

Creamy Veggie Bake

1 package silken, firm tofu
1/2 cup cashew cream   (Blend 1/4 cup cashew bits in 1/2 cup water
  until smooth.)
2 tablespoons Dijon mustard
3 tablespoons grated soy Parmesan
1 teaspoon Herbamare
1 red pepper, chopped
1 small onion, diced
1 green pepper, chopped
1 zucchini, chopped
4 cups broccoli florets
1 tablespoon olive oil
1 1/2 cups shredded cheddar soy cheese

1. Heat oven to 350 degrees.
2. In a processor, cream the tofu, cashew cream, mustard, Parmesan and Herbamare.
3. In a dutch oven, sauté the peppers, onion and zucchini in the oil for about 10 minutes. Remove from heat.
4. Add the broccoli, soy cheese, and tofu mixture and stir everything together, mixing well.
5. Bake for about 40 minutes.

Serves 4 to 6.

Curried Tofu

1 tub of Chinese-style, firm tofu, sliced, frozen, then thawed and
    squeezed to remove water
1/8 cup grated fresh ginger
1 teaspoon minced garlic
1/8 cup water
2 tablespoons almond butter
1 tablespoon tamari
1 1/2 teaspoons curry powder
Dash of cayenne
1 tablespoon sesame oil
1 medium onion, minced
2 cups almond milk
1/2 teaspoon salt
1 package frozen green peas, thawed in a colander under hot
    running water
1/2 cup toasted almonds

1. Cut tofu in to thin strips. Set aside.
2. Combine ginger, garlic, water, almond butter, tamari, curry powder, and cayenne in a food processor and process until thoroughly blended.
3. Pour mixture over tofu strips and gently turn and press until tofu has absorbed the mixture.
4. In a large skillet, sauté the onion in oil for about 5 minutes.
5. Add tofu and continue to cook until tofu starts to brown.
6. Add almond milk, salt, and peas.
7. Bring to a simmer and cook for about 2 minutes.
8. Remove from heat and stir in almonds.

Serves 4 to 6.

Grilled Tofu Steaks

1 tub Chinese-style firm tofu, pressed
3 tablespoons tamari
1/4 cup dry white wine
2 teaspoons minced garlic
1/2 teaspoon coriander
1/2 teaspoon marjoram
2 tablespoons grapeseed oil

1. Cut tofu into 1/2 inch thick slices
2. Combine tamari, wine, garlic, coriander, and marjoram and marinate tofu for at least 1 hour (preferably 2), in the refrigerator, turning once.
3. Brush tofu with the oil and grill outdoors or under the broiler until slightly brown on both sides.

Serves 6.

Tofu Loaf

1 teaspoon olive oil
1/2 medium-size onion, diced
10 medium mushrooms, diced
3 teaspoons minced garlic
5 tablespoons tahini
1/2 cup pecans
1/2 cup toasted almonds
1/2 cup hulled sesame seeds
2 tablespoons Vogue Vege Base
1 1/2 teaspoons sea salt
1/8 teaspoon cayenne
1/2 teaspoon each: basil, oregano, kelp, and savory
1 tub Chinese-style firm tofu, pressed
1 egg, beaten

1. Heat oven to 350 degrees and spray glass loaf pan with oil.
2. Sauté the onion in the oil for 2 minutes.
3. Add the mushrooms and sauté for 4 more minutes, then add garlic, cover, and cook for 3 more minutes.
4. Stir in tahini and remove from heat.
5. Combine nuts in a food processor and process to a coarse meal.
6. Put nuts into a bowl and add sesame seeds, Vege Base, and all the seasonings. Mix well.
7. Crumble the tofu and stir into the onion tahini mixture.
8. Add the beaten egg to the dry mixture, then add the tofu mixture, mixing well.
9. Form into a loaf and put into loaf pan. Bake for 1 hour.

While the loaf is baking, make a sauce using:

1 teaspoon olive oil
1/2 onion, diced
1 teaspoon minced garlic
2 14.5-ounce cans organic diced tomatoes
2 teaspoons tamari
1 teaspoon basil
1 teaspoon Herbamare

1. Sauté onion in oil for 5 minutes. Add the garlic and sauté 2 minutes.
2. Add the rest of the ingredients, cover and simmer for 30 minutes.
3. Remove the cover and simmer for 15 more minutes.

Remove the loaf from the oven and let cool for 10 to 15 minutes. Slice into individual servings covered with the sauce.

Serves 6 to 8.

Tofu-Cauliflower Casserole

2 cups cauliflower, chopped
1/2 medium-sized onion, diced
1/2 green pepper, diced
1 tablespoon olive oil
1 package silken, firm tofu
1 tablespoon soy sauce
1 cup grated soy cheese
1/4 teaspoon curry powder
1 teaspoon sea salt
dash of cayenne and kelp

1. Heat oven to 350 degrees and spray an oven proof casserole dish with oil.
2. Steam cauliflower until tender. (About 8 minutes)
3. Sauté onion and pepper in the oil.
4. In a food processor, cream tofu. Then add the next 6 ingredients and process until thoroughly mixed.
5 Transfer to a bowl and stir in the cauliflower and the onion mixture.
6. Bake for 35 to 40 minutes.

Serves 4.

Szechuan Tofu and Stir-Fried Vegetables

1 tub Chinese-style firm tofu, pressed and cut into 1-inch cubes
3 tablespoons tamari
2 cups water
1 6-ounce can tomato paste
2 tablespoons lime juice
2 teaspoons fresh grated ginger
2 teaspoons garlic powder
1/2 teaspoon Tobasco
3 tablespoons kudzu dissolved in 1/4 cup water
1 tablespoon grapeseed oil
1 cup onions, cut into half-moons
1/2 cup matchstick carrots
1 cup sliced celery
1 green pepper, chopped
3 cups snow peas, strings removed

1. Marinate the tofu in the tamari for 30 minutes.
2. Place tofu on an oiled baking sheet and bake at 350 degrees for 30 minutes.
3. To make the sauce, combine the water and the next 5 ingredients in a saucepan. Bring to a boil, stir in the kudzu-water mixture, and simmer until thickened. Then remove from heat.
4. Meanwhile, in a wok or large skillet, stir fry the vegetables in the oil, starting with the onion, then the carrots, then the other vegetables, holding out the snow peas until the last minute.
5. Stir in the tofu and the sauce.

Serves 6.

ACID-PROTEIN EGG DISHES

Egg Replacer Silken Omelet

Filling:
5 ounces silken, firm tofu (1/2 package)
2 teaspoons olive oil
1/4 teaspoon salt
1 tablespoon lemon juice
1/2 teaspoon dried, minced onion
3 or 4 dashes cayenne
2 green onions, minced
1/4 cup red pepper, minced
Omelet:
1/2 cup egg replacer for each omelete
Soy Parmesan
Paprika

1. In a food processor, combine tofu, oil, salt, lemon juice, dried onion and cayenne. Process until smooth and creamy. (Scrape down once.)
2. Add green onion and red pepper and pulse just until blended.
3. Turn on oven broiler.
4. Assemble egg replacer, non-stick skillet, olive oil (optional), paprika and soy Parmesan.
5. Heat skillet, medium-low heat. Pour a tiny amount of olive oil in the center of the skillet then slowly pour the egg replacer (for one omelete) into the center of the oil.
6. Cook until the edges of the omelet are done and transfer skillet to the oven broiler. Watch carefully and remove when the top of the omelete is firm.
7. Transfer omelete to a plate and spread one-fourth of the tofu mixture down the center of the omelete. Fold omelete over and sprinkle with soy parmesan and paprika.
8. Repeat for each omelete. (Makes up to 4.)

Good served with a mound of finely grated cole slaw on top of a slice of tomato.

Basic Omelet For Two

2 eggs, beaten
1/2 package silken tofu, firm, mashed
1/2 teaspoon Herbamare
dash of cayenne

1. Whisk eggs, tofu, and seasonings together.
2. Pour into an oiled skillet and cook on low heat until bottom of omelet is set. Meanwhile, turn on oven broiler.
3. Place skillet under broiler and cook until top is set.
4. Transfer omelet to a dish. Spoon filling of choice on top of omelet and fold over. Serve hot.

Variations on Basic Omelet

Mushroom omelet - Add 1/2 cup of sautéed mushrooms to omelet before cooking.

Herbed omelet - Add 1 tablespoon minced parsley, 1/4 teaspoon garlic powder, 1/4 teaspoon chervil, and chopped chives or scallions to taste.

Fresh herb omelet - Add minced parsley and any other fresh herbs that are available, minced. Include chives or scallions.

Soy cheese omelet - Grate soy cheese of any variety and add to the top of the omelet before folding. Add Worcestershire sauce to the cheese for a different flavor.

Other fillings for omelets - Chopped, sautéed spinach; creamed asparagus; sautéed or steamed broccoli with grated soy cheese; any leftover or canned seafood, creamed; any vegetable you especially like, snowpeas, English peas, or what-have-you.

Spanish Omelet Sauce

1/2 large onion, chopped
1/2 green bell pepper, cut in strips
2 small stalks celery, chopped
2 teaspoons grapeseed oil
6 stuffed olives, sliced
1 14.5-ounce can diced, organic tomatoes
4 to 6 slices pickled jalapeños, minced
Herbamare to taste
1/2 cup grated soy cheddar (optional)

1. In a sauce pan, sauté onion, pepper, and celery in the oil until semi-soft.
2. Add the rest of the ingredients except the soy cheese, bring to a boil, lower heat and simmer, uncovered, for about 20 minutes.
3. Spoon some of the mixture on top of omelets before folding them and spoon the rest on the folded top. Add the optional cheese before folding.

Serves 4.

Vegetable Omelet

1/2 medium onion, diced
1 stalk celery, diced
1/4 cup sliced mushrooms
1/4 green bell pepper, diced
1/4 red bell pepper, diced
2 teaspoons oil
4 cherry tomatoes, sliced
2 scallions, chopped
2 eggs, beaten
1/2 package silken tofu, firm, mashed
2 teaspoons tamari
1/2 cup grated soy cheddar

1. Sauté onion, celery, mushrooms and peppers in oil in a large skillet for about 5 minutes, until semi-soft. Remove from skillet and set aside.
2. Combine eggs, tofu, and tamari and pour into the skillet. Turn oven broiler on.
3. When eggs have set on the bottom, slide skillet under the broiler and cook until top is firm. Sprinkle cheese on top of eggs during the last minute.
4. Divide omelet in half and put on plates. Divide vegetable mixture and spoon on omelets then fold.
5. Garnish tops with sliced tomatoes and scallions. Serve hot.

Serves 2.

For a spicier omelet, you can add 1/2 cup of salsa to the vegetable mixture.

Scrambled Eggs

Whisk eggs, tofu and seasonings together as in the basic omelet. Cook over low heat, stirring and turning occasionally. Cook until just set.

A great many herbs or lightly steamed or sautéed vegetables can be added to scrambled eggs. For example, steamed asparagus tips, broccoli or zucchini; sautéed cauliflower, spinach, celery, bell peppers, or onions.

Use your imagination. Lots of herbs can be successfully combined with eggs.

Deviled Eggs

6 firm-cooked eggs
1/4 package of silken tofu, firm
2 teaspoons cider vinegar
2 teaspoons prepared mustard
3 tablespoons mayonnaise
1/4 teaspoon cayenne
1/4 teaspoon Herbamare

1. Cut eggs in half, remove yolks. Put 2 of the yolks and the tofu into a bowl and mash. (Discard the other yolks.)
2. Mix the yolk mixture with the rest of the ingredients, stirring until smooth.
3. Stuff the yolk mixture back into the whites. Garnish with paprika. Chill.

Serves 6.

Zucchini Pancake

2 cups grated zucchini
1/2 cup grated onion
1/2 cup grated soy mozzarella
1/3 cup soy Parmesan
1/3 cup pecans or walnuts ground into a meal in a processor
1/2 teaspoon Herbamare
2 egg whites, beaten until frothy

1. Heat oven to 400 degrees and oil a 9" x 11" baking dish.
2. Place zucchini and onion in a colander and press to squeeze out excess juice.
3. In a bowl, combine all but the egg whites and mix well. Add egg whites and stir until well blended.
4. Pour into baking dish, spread evenly.
5. Bake for 30 to 40 minutes, until golden brown. Serve hot.

Serves 2.

ACID-PROTEIN SEAFOOD

Fish Dijon

1 large sweet onion, diced
1 tablespoon olive oil
1 teaspoon dried dill
1 1/2 cups almond milk
3 tablespoons Dijon mustard
1 teaspoon Herbamare
1 1/2 tablespoons arrowroot dissolved in 1/8 cup of water
1 tablespoon lemon juice
2 pounds fish fillets

1. In a large skillet, sauté onion and dill in oil for 5 minutes.
2. Meanwhile, in a blender, purée the cashews in half of the almond milk until smooth. Add the rest of the milk, the Dijon mustard, the Herbamare, and the arrowroot mixture and blend until mixed. Add to the onion mixture.
3. Place fish on a baking dish and broil until opaque.
4. Meanwhile, simmer sauce until creamy and thick. Stir in the lemon juice.
5. Pour sauce over the broiled fish.

Serves 4.

Fish Fromage

1 onion, diced
1/2 package soy cheddar cheese, grated
2 pounds orange roughy or other white fish
2 tablespoons Worcestershire sauce
2 teaspoons prepared mustard
1/2 teaspoon sea salt
few dashes cayenne
1 cup almond milk

1. Heat oven to 425 degrees.
2. Spread onion and half of the cheese on the bottom of a baking dish. Place the fish on top.
3. Combine the remaining ingredients and pour over the fish. Sprinkle the rest of the cheese on top.
4. Bake for 30 minutes.

Serves 4.

Fish With Artichokes

1 large sweet onion, diced
2 teaspoons minced garlic
2 cups sliced mushrooms
1 tablespoon olive oil
1/2 teaspoon each: basil and oregano
1/8 cup fresh lemon juice
1/4 cup dry white wine
1 teaspoon Herbamare
1 teaspoon arrowroot dissolved in 1 tablespoon of water
2 pounds white fish fillets
1 18-ounce can artichoke hearts, drained and halved

1. Heat oven to 350 degrees.
2. In a large skillet, sauté the onions, garlic, and mushrooms in the oil for 5 minutes.
3. Stir in the herbs. Continue cooking until the mushrooms begin to brown, then stir in the lemon juice, wine, Herbamare, and arrowroot.
4. Place fish in an oiled baking dish, top with the artichoke hearts, and pour the sauce over all.
5. Bake, covered for 20 minutes. Uncover and bake until the fish flakes easily with a fork.

Serves 4.

Baked Whitefish With Horseradish-Mayonnaise

2 pounds of white fish fillets
1/2 cup light mayonnaise
1/4 cup prepared horseradish

1. Heat oven to 400 degrees.
2. Combine mayonnaise and horseradish, spread over the fish.
3. Bake fish for about 15 minutes, until opaque and flakes easily with a fork.

Serves 4.

Broiled Fish With Almond Pesto

2 pounds white fish fillets
1 cup blanched almonds
2 tablespoons minced garlic
1/2 cup olive oil
1/8 cup dry white wine
1 teaspoon salt
1/2 teaspoon cayenne pepper
1 teaspoon paprika

1. Heat oven to 350 degrees.
2. Spread almonds on baking sheet and roast for 5 to 10 minutes, until they start to turn a golden brown. Let cool completely.
3. Combine the garlic, olive oil, wine, salt, cayenne, and paprika.
4. Broil fish for about 10 minutes, until it flakes easily with a fork.
5. Chop the toasted almonds into small pieces (or pulse briefly in processor).
6. Add almonds to the other ingredients and mix well.
7. Top each fillet with pesto. Serve immediately.

Serves 4.

Grilled Tuna With Teriyaki Sauce

This is our favorite dish, served over a Romaine salad with an olive oil-balsamic vinegar dressing. Garnish with Niçoise or Kalamata olives, celery sticks, and halved cherry tomatoes.

2 pounds of tuna steaks

Marinade:
1/3 cup tamari
1/3 cup grapeseed oil
1 teaspoon minced garlic
1 tablespoon fresh grated ginger
1/3 cup dry sherry

1. Combine the marinade ingredients. Rinse the tuna steaks, puncture the surface a number of times with a fork, and put in a baking dish. Pour the marinade over the fish and chill for about 30 minutes.
2. Grill the fish over hot coals, basting occasionally with the marinade.

Serves 4.

Shrimp Creole

1/2 sweet onion, diced
1/2 green bell pepper, diced
1/2 cup chopped mushrooms
1 tablespoon oil
1 14.5-ounce can diced organic tomatoes
1/4 cup sliced, stuffed olives
1/2 teaspoon Herbamare
1/2 teaspoon cayenne
1/8 cup dry sherry (optional)
2 pounds cooked, peeled shrimp
2 cups diced zucchini

1. In a large saucepan, sauté onion, pepper, and mushroom in oil for about 10 minutes.
2. Add tomatoes, olives, seasonings, and sherry and cook for 5 more minutes.
3. Add zucchini and cook 2 more minutes.
4. Add shrimp and simmer until heated.

Serves 4.

Crab and Mushroom Bake

10 medium button mushrooms, chopped
1 tablespoon oil
2 teaspoons Vogue Vege Base
1 1/2 tablespoons kudzu
1 1/2 cups water
1/4 teaspoons each: basil, savory, and celery salt
1 6-ounce can crab meat
1 large avocado, cubed
2 tablespoons minced pimento
1/2 cup grated soy cheddar cheese

1. Heat oven to 350 degrees.
2. In a large skillet, sauté mushrooms in oil for about 8 minutes. Stir in Vege Base.
3. Dissolve kudzu in the water and stir into the mushroom mixture. Add the other seasonings and cook, stirring until the mixture thickens.
4. Add the drained crab, avocado, and pimento and spoon into 2 oiled, individual baking dishes.
5. Top with soy cheese and bake for 20 minutes.

Serves 2.

Deviled Crab

2 egg whites
2 tablespoons tomato sauce
2 teaspoons Pickapeppa sauce
1 teaspoon Dijon mustard
1 red pepper minced
1/2 teaspoon salt
1 6-ounce can crab meat, drained
1/2 cup coarsely chopped almonds

1. Heat oven to 350 degrees.
2. Combine egg whites with white sauce, tomato sauce, Pickapeppa, mustard, bell pepper, salt, and crab meat.
3. Pour into 2 oiled, individual baking dishes and bake for 15 minutes.
4. Remove from oven, sprinkle top with the almonds and bake another 7 to 10 minutes. Watch carefully so that the nuts don't burn. They should just be a golden color.

Serves 2.

Barbecued Salmon

1 large salmon fillet

Sauce:
1 onion, diced
1/2 cup celery, diced
1 tablespoon oil
2 tablespoons apple cider vinegar
2 tablespoons balsamic vinegar
1 cup tomato sauce
3 tablespoons Worcestershire sauce
1 teaspoon prepared mustard
1/2 cup water
10 drops stevia (or to taste)
1/2 teaspoon salt
1/2 teaspoon cayenne

1. Sauté onion and celery in oil for 5 minutes. Add the rest of the sauce ingredients and simmer for 30 minutes.
2. Transfer to blender and purée.
3. Pour sauce on the salmon fillet and grill, skin side down, over hot coals for about 20 minutes, basting with the barbeque sauce occasionally.

Serves 4 to 6.

Shrimp-Cashew Szechuan Stir Fry

1 tablespoon oil
1/2 large onion, chopped
1 carrot, cut in matchsticks
1 green bell pepper, sliced
2 cups small broccoli florets
20 snow peas, strings removed
2 scallions, chopped
3/4 cup oven-roasted cashews
1 1/4 pounds cooked shrimp

Sauce:
1/8 cup tamari
1/2 teaspoon Szechuan sauce
6 drops stevia (or to taste)
1/8 cup dry sherry
1 teaspoon kudzu dissolved in 1 tablespoon water

1. Combine sauce ingredients. Set aside.
2. In a large wok, cook onion in oil for 2 minutes. Add carrots and cook 1 more minute. Add pepper, broccoli, and snow peas and cook 1 more minute.
3. Add cashews and shrimp and stir in the sauce. Cook just until heated through

Serves 4.

Tuna Casserole

1 cup almond milk
1/4 cup cashew pieces
1/2 teaspoon minced garlic
1/2 teaspoon dill
1 teaspoon Dijon mustard
2 teaspoons lemon juice
1 6-ounce can solid white tuna
1 can artichoke hearts, drained and chopped
1/4 cup sliced, stuffed green olives
1 zucchini, chopped

1. Heat oven to 350 degrees.
2. In a blender, purée the cashews in the almond milk. Add the next 4 ingredients and blend.
3. Drain tuna and break into small bits.
4. Put tuna, cashew mixture, artichokes, olives, and zucchini in a bowl and mix well.
5. Pour into an oiled baking dish and bake for 30 minutes.

Serves 2.

Salmon Patties With Mustard Sauce

1 16-ounce can red salmon or 1 lb. cooked fresh
1 egg white
2 tablespoons lemon juice
1 teaspoon dried dill
1/4 cup soy powder
1 tablespoon olive oil

1. Drain salmon. Remove skin and bones.
2. Beat together the egg white, lemon juice, and dill. Then beat in the soy powder.
3. Stir the egg mixture into the salmon, breaking salmon into small pieces.
4. Form into patties and fry in the oil over medium heat. Brown both sides.
5. Meanwhile, make the Mustard Sauce.

Mustard Sauce:
1/2 cup pure water
1 tablespoon apple cider vinegar
1 teaspoon prepared horseradish
1 tablespoon prepared mustard
1 teaspoon arrowroot dissolved in 1 tablespoon water

1. Heat water, vinegar, horseradish, and mustard in a small saucepan.
2. Add dissolved arrowroot. Simmer until slightly thick.
3. Pour over salmon patties. Garnish with paprika or minced parsley.

Serves 2.

Poached Fish With Mushrooms

4 small fish fillets
1/2 sweet onion, diced
1/4 cup fresh, minced parsley
2 cups chopped mushrooms
1 tablespoon oil
1/2 cup dry white wine
1/4 cup pure water
1 tablespoon arrowroot, dissolved in 1 tablespoon water

1. In a large skillet, sauté the onion, parsley, and mushrooms in the oil for about 10 minutes.
2. Add wine and water, stirring to mix.
3. Lay fillets in skillet, cover and poach for 10 minutes. Remove to plate.
4. Thicken sauce with arrowroot. Pour over fish. Sprinkle with paprika.

Serves 4.

Canned Tuna-Bake

1 9-ounce can solid white albacore tuna packed in water
1/4 cup chopped scallions
1/3 cup light mayonnaise
1 tablespoon fresh lemon juice
1/8 teaspoon cayenne

1. Heat oven to 350 degrees and spray 2 individual baking dishes with oil.
2. Mix all ingredients together, breaking tuna into small pieces.
3. Spoon into the oiled dishes and bake for 30 minutes.

This recipe is so easy and really very good! It's great to fix for an emergency meal.

Serves 2.

ACID-PROTEIN VEGETABLES

Savory Brussels Sprouts

2 cups of water
12 Brussels sprouts
2 teaspoon balsamic vinegar
2 teaspoon lemon zest
1 tablespoon lemon juice
1 tablespoon olive oil
sea salt and cayenne to taste

1. In a large saucepan, bring water to a boil and add Brussels sprouts. Cover and cook about 8 minutes, until just barely tender.
2. Meanwhile, whisk together the rest of the ingredients in a small bowl.
3. Drain the sprouts and transfer to a serving bowl. Toss with the vinegar mixture.

Serves 4.

Zucchini with Ginger and Cashews

4 small zucchini
1 carrot
2 tablespoons grapeseed oil
1 teaspoon grated ginger
1/2 teaspoon minced garlic
1/4 teaspoon sea salt
1/3 cup chopped, roasted cashews

1. Cut each zucchini in half, length-wise, and then into 1/4-inch thick slices. Cut the carrot with a vegetable peeler, for paper-thin slices.
2. Heat oil in a wok, add vegetables, ginger, garlic, and salt. Cook about 3 minutes, stir in cashews, and serve.

Serves 4.

Mushroom-Zucchini Puff

1 1/2 cups sliced mushrooms
1 teaspoon olive oil
2 1/2 cups shredded zucchini, squeezed to remove liquid
1/2 cup sliced scallions
2 large egg whites, beaten 'til frothy
5 drops stevia
1 tablespoon orange zest
2 teaspoons grated ginger
1/4 teaspoon nutmeg
1/2 teaspoon salt

1. Heat oven to 350 degrees.
2. Oil a 2-quart baking dish.
3. In a skillet, sauté the mushrooms in the oil for about 5 minutes.
4. Combine the egg, stevia, zest, ginger, nutmeg, and salt in a bowl. Add the vegetables and mushrooms and mix well.
5. Pour into the baking dish and bake for 45 minutes to an hour or until puffed and golden. (A knife inserted comes out clean.)

Serves 4.

Zucchini with Fresh Basil

1 tablespoon olive oil
1 1/2 teaspoons minced garlic
1/2 large, sweet onion, minced
3 plum tomatoes, diced
2 cups zucchini, sliced
1/2 cup red bell pepper, minced
2 tablespoons fresh basil, minced
1/8 cup white wine

1. In a large skillet, heat oil and sauté the onion 3 minutes. Add all but the basil and wine and cover. Cook about 5 minutes.
2. Uncover, add basil and wine, and cook for 3 more minutes.

Serves 4.

Puréed Eggplant

1 small eggplant
2 tablespoons lemon juice
1 teaspoon minced garlic
2 teaspoons dark sesame oil
1/2 teaspoon curry powder
2 teaspoons tamari

1. Heat oven to 400 degrees.
2. Slice eggplant in half, lengthwise and lightly salt. Leave for 15 minutes and allow to sweat. Blot off water and salt with a paper towel.
3. Place eggplant on a baking sheet, cut side down and bake for 30 minutes.
4. Remove from oven, allow to cool slightly and skin. Chop eggplant flesh and combine with other ingredients in a food processor. Purée until smooth.

Serves 4.

Broccoli-Red Pepper Stir-Fry

1 tablespoon grapeseed oil
1/2 large, sweet onion, chopped
2 teaspoons minced garlic
2 teaspoons grated ginger
1 head of small broccoli florets
1 red bell pepper, sliced
1/8 cup white wine
1 teaspoon tamari
1 teaspoon dark sesame oil
2 tablespoons sesame seeds, toasted*

1. In a wok or large skillet, heat oil, add onion, and sauté for 3 minutes.
2. Add garlic and ginger and stir-fry for 15 seconds.
3. Add the broccoli and pepper, stirring and tossing to mix well.
4. Add the wine and cover. Cook for 2 minutes.
5. Remove cover and cook on high heat just until the vegetables are tender-crisp.
6. Add soy sauce and sesame oil and remove from heat. Stir to mix well.
7. Sprinkle sesame seeds over all.

Serves 4.

* To toast, stir seeds in a dry skillet over medium heat until golden and fragrent.

Green Beans Almondine

1/2 cup blanched, toasted almonds*
1 teaspoon oil
1 teaspoon minced garlic
1 pound green beans, trimmed and chopped
1/8 cup dry white wine
2 tablespoons lemon juice
1/4 teaspoon Herbamare
1 teaspoon dark sesame oil

1. Heat oil in wok or skillet and add garlic. Stir for a few seconds and add the green beans. Add the wine and cover. Cook about 5 minutes, or until the greenbeans are bright green and crisp-tender.
2. Meanwhile, whisk together the lemon juice, Herbamare, and sesame oil.
3. When beans are done, toss with the lemon juice mixture and the almonds.

Serves 4.

*Spread blanched almonds on a baking sheet and bake at 350 degrees for 8 to 10 minutes. Watch carefully, they brown quickly.

Cauliflower with Peanut Sauce

1/4 cup natural peanut butter
1/8 cup lemon juice
1/8 cup pure water
1/2 teaspoon minced garlic
1/3 cup fresh, minced parsley
1/2 teaspoon Herbamare
dash of kelp
1/8 teaspoon cayenne
1 small head of cauliflower, chopped
1 red bell pepper, diced
1/2 cup water

1. Whisk together the first 8 ingredients (reserving some of the parsley for garnish). Set aside.
2. In a large skillet, heat water, add cauliflower and bell pepper, cover. Bring to a boil, lower heat, and simmer for about 15 minutes. Remove cover and simmer until water evaporates.
3. Remove from heat and stir in sauce.
4. Garnish with reserved parsley.

Serves 4.

Broccoli Casserole

4 cups small broccoli florets
2 egg whites
2 cups chopped button mushrooms
1 1/2 cups almond milk, blended with 1/4 cup raw cashew pieces
1 teaspoon Herbamare
1/8 teaspoon cayenne
1/2 large sweet onion, diced
2 cups shredded soy cheddar

1. Heat oven to 350 degrees. Oil a 2-quart baking dish.
2. Put broccoli in baking dish. Combine the rest of the ingredients, except soy cheese, and pour over the broccoli. Sprinkle the cheese over the top.
3. Bake for about 30 minutes.

Serves 4.

Stuffed Zucchini

4 large zucchini
2 teaspoons olive oil
1/2 cup shredded yellow squash
1/4 cup chopped scallions
1/3 cup finely chopped pecans
1/2 teaspoon Herbamare
1 cup chopped cheddar soy cheese
1 tablespoon Worcestershire sauce
1 tablespoon lemon juice
1/2 teaspoon dried basil

1. Heat oven to 350 degrees and spray a 9"x13" baking dish.
2. Slice the zucchini lengthwise in halves. Scoop out most of the pulp, leaving 1/4-inch shells. Dice the pulp.
3. In a skillet, sauté the yellow squash and diced zucchini in the oil for 3 or 4 minutes.
4. Add the scallions and nuts. Remove from heat.
5. Combine the Herbamare, soy, cheddar, Worcestershire sauce, lemon juice, and basil in a food processor and process until creamy.
6. Stir the soy cheese mixture into the vegetable mixture and stuff the zucchini shells.
7. Place stuffed zucchini in the baking dish and bake for 30 minutes.

Serves 8.

ACID-PROTEIN SAUCES AND GRAVIES

Cashew Sauce

2 cups water
1/2 cup cashews
2 tablespoons onion flakes
1 1/2 teaspoons Herbamare
1/2 cup dry sherry
1 teaspoon arrowroot
1/8 cup cold water

1. Blend cashews and water in a blender until smooth.
2. Put in a saucepan with the onion flakes, Herbamare, and sherry and bring to a simmer.
3. Dissolve the arrowroot in the cold water and stir into the sauce. Heat until thickened.

Almond Ginger Sauce

1 cup blanched almonds
1/3 cup roasted, blanched almonds
2 cups pure water
2 teaspoons Vogue Vege Base
1 teaspoon minced garlic
1 tablespoon fresh, grated ginger
1 tablespoon tamari
1 1/2 tablespoons lemon juice
1/4 teaspoon cayenne

Blend all ingredients until smooth.

Good on steamed vegetables or as a dip.

Jalapeño-Dill Sauce

1 package silken tofu, firm
1 tablespoon grapeseed oil
6 slices pickled jalapeño, minced
1/2 teaspoon minced garlic
1 teaspoon dill weed
1 tablespoon lemon juice
1/2 teaspoon tamari

Blend all ingredients until smooth.

Good on vegetables or as a salad dressing.

Peanut Sauce

1 large, sweet onion, chopped
1 teaspoon minced garlic
2 teaspoons grapeseed oil
1/2 cup natural peanut butter
1 tablespoon dark sesame oil
3 tablespoons tamari
2 tablespoons cumin
2 tablespoons ground ginger
1/4 teaspoon cayenne
6 drops stevia
1 1/2 cups water
2 teaspoons Vogue Vege Base

1. In a skillet, sauté onions and garlic in the grapeseed oil for 8 minutes.
2. Transfer to a blender and add the remaining ingredients, blending until smooth.
3. Return to the skillet and bring to a boil, lower heat and simmer 2 minutes.

Good on tempeh, baked tofu, or vegetables.

Lemon Sauce

1/2 package silken tofu, firm
2 tablespoons fresh lemon juice
1 tablespoon white balsamic vinegar
few drops of stevia, to taste
1/2 teaspoon salt
dash cayenne
water to thin, as needed

Purée in a processor until smooth. Use on steamed vegetables or as a dip for artichokes.

Soy Cheese Sauce

1/3 cup raw cashew pieces
2 cups water
1/2 package Soya Kaas cheddar cheese cut in small pieces
2 teaspoons Dijon mustard
1/2 teaspoon salt
1/4 teaspoon cayenne

1. Blend cashew pieces in 1 cup of water until smooth.
2. Add the rest of the ingredients and blend until smooth.
3. Heat, stirring, in a saucepan.

Especially good on asparagus or cauliflower.

Cashew-Ginger Sauce

1 1/2 cups toasted cashews
3/4 cup water
2 tablespoons grated ginger
1 tablespoon tamari
2 tablespoons cider vinegar
5 drops stevia
1/2 teaspoon salt
1/4 teaspoon cayenne

1. Purée all ingredients in a processor.
2. Transfer to a saucepan and gently heat.

Great on steamed broccoli or baked vegetables.

Sweet and Sour Sauce

1/2 sweet onion, quartered and sliced
1/4 cup carrots, cut in matchsticks
1/3 cup red bell pepper slices
1 tablespoon grapeseed oil
1 cup water
1 teaspoon Vogue Vege Base
1 tablespoon tamari
1 tablespoon cider vinegar
1 1/2 teaspoons grated ginger
1 teaspoon minced garlic
8 drops stevia
1 tablespoon arrowroot dissolved in 1 tablespoon water

1. Sauté onion and carrot in oil for 5 minutes. Add pepper and cook 2 more minutes.
2. Combine the rest of the ingredients in the skillet and stir in the arrowroot. Stir until thickened.

Barbecue Sauce

2 tablespoons Heinz Light Catsup
1 tablespoon Worcestershire sauce
1 tablespoon Dijon mustard
2 tablespoons minced onion
2 teaspoons minced garlic
1/4 cup dry red wine
dash of liquid smoke
several drops of stevia, to taste
Tobasco to taste

Combine all ingredients and brush on fish, tofu, or tempeh. Grill.

Roasted Pecan Gravy

2/3 cup pecans, oven-roasted
1 10.5-ounce package silken tofu, firm
1 tablespoon grapeseed oil
1 onion, chopped
2 small stalks celery, chopped
1/8 cup dry sherry
1 tablespoon lemon juice
1 teaspoon minced garlic
2 teaspoons Bragg's amino acids
Water as needed

1. Grind pecans in a processor to a fine meal, crumble in tofu and purée.
2 In a skillet, sauté onion and celery in the oil for 5 minutes. Add the sherry, lemon juice, garlic, and amino acids and simmer for 2 minutes.
3. Transfer skillet ingredients to the food processor and process with the pecan-tofu mixture until it is smooth, adding water to get a gravy-like consistency.
4. Pour gravy back into the skillet and heat gently before serving.

Good over tofu, tempeh, or vegetables.

PROTEIN-ACID DESSERTS

Butterscotch Mousse with Toasted Almonds

2 heaping tablespoons raw cashew pieces
2 teaspoons butterscotch flavor
1/8 teaspoon vanilla
2 teaspoons pure water
1/3 package silken tofu, extra-firm
8 to 10 drops of stevia, or to taste
1 tablespoons chopped, toasted almonds

1. In a processor, process cashews until they are a very fine meal.
2. Add the next 5 ingredients and process until the mixture is smooth and creamy.
3. Spoon into 2 small dessert cups. Refrigerate for an hour or so to let flavors blend.
4. Sprinkle 1 tablespoon of almonds on top of each dessert just before serving.

Serves 2.

Lemon Mousse

2 heaping tablespoons raw cashew bits
2 tablespoons fresh lemon juice
1/8 teaspoon vanilla
10 to 12 drops of stevia, or to taste
1/3 package of silken tofu, extra-firm
1 teaspoon grated lemon rind

1. In a processor, process cashews until they are a very fine meal.
2. Add the rest of the ingredients except the lemon rind and process until the mixture is smooth and creamy.
3. Add the lemon rind and pulse until well mixed.
4. Spoon into 2 small dessert cups and refrigerate for an hour or 2 to let the flavors meld.
5. Garnish with paper-thin slice of lemon.

Serves 2.

Mocha Mousse with Toasted Pecans

Prepare Teccino liquid by putting 2 heaping tablespoons Teccino Chocolate Mint in a cup. Add 1/4 cup boiling water. Steep for 5 minutes. Strain through a coffee filter.

2 heaping tablespoons cashew pieces
1/3 package of silken tofu, extra-firm
1 1/2 tablespoons Teccino liquid
1/8 teaspoon vanilla
8 to 10 drops of stevia, or to taste
2 tablespoons toasted, chopped pecans

1. In a food processor, process the cashews into a very fine meal.
2. Add the rest of the ingredients except the pecans and process until the mixture is smooth and creamy.
3. Spoon into 2 small dessert cups and refrigerate for an hour or so to let flavors meld.
4. Just before serving sprinkle 1 tablespoon pecans on top of each.

Serves 2.

NEUTRAL APPETIZERS

The best appetizer of all is a large plate of crisp raw vegetables. I use carrot sticks, celery sticks, jicama, cucumber slices, zucchini or yellow squash, broccoli and cauliflower florets, cherry tomatoes, and red pepper slices. (I, personally, like to steam the broccoli for about 3 minutes then rinse with cold water and pat dry. It is prettier and easier to digest than raw broccoli.)

Since everyone seems to want to dip the vegetables in something, here is a great neutral dip.

Roasted Red Pepper Dip

6 red bell peppers, roasted and peeled (or a large jar of roasted peppers)
3 tablespoons olive oil
3 tablespoons balsamic vinegar
3 or 4 drops stevia

In a processor, purée all ingredients until smooth.

Of course, if you are having an acid-protein meal, you can use any of the acid dips with the neutral vegetables or use the alkaline-starch dips if you are serving a starch meal.

NEUTRAL SOUPS

Neutral Gazpacho

2 ripe, organic tomatoes, chopped
1 small cucumber, peeled, seeded and chopped (If organic, don't peel)
1/2 bell pepper, (red or green) chopped
1/2 small onion, peeled and chopped
1 tablespoon balsamic vinegar
1 teaspoon Vogue Vege Base
1 cup ice water
1 teaspoon Herbamare
dash tobasco

Put all the ingredients in a blender and purée. Leave some texture or blend until smooth.

Serves 2.

Vegetable Soup

1 tablespoon olive oil
1 large onion, diced
4 stalks celery, diced
4 carrots, scrubbed and sliced
3 tablespoons Vogue Vege Base
2 quarts water
1/2 small head green cabbage, shredded
4 leaves kale, stem removed, shredded
1/4 pound fresh green beans, trimmed and chopped into
    1" pieces
2 zucchini, chopped
4 small yellow squash, chopped
dash cayenne and kelp
1 1/2 tablespoons fines herbs
sea salt to taste

1. In a soup pot, sauté onion, celery, and carrots in oil for 5 minutes.
2. Stir in Vege Base, add water and all the vegetables except the zucchini and yellow squash.
3. Bring to a boil, cover, lower heat and simmer for 30 minutes.
4. Add zucchini, yellow squash, cayenne, kelp, fines herbs, and a pinch of sea salt. Simmer another 15 minutes.
5. Season to taste and serve.

Quick Steamed Vegetable Soup

1 large carrot, scrubbed and sliced thin
1 stalk celery, chopped
1 small onion, sliced
1 small wedge green cabbage, chopped
1 tablespoon Vogue Vege Base
1/2 teaspoon sea salt
dash each, kelp and cayenne
2 1/2 cups boiling water plus water from steaming vegetables

1. Steam the vegetables for about 10 minutes, until the carrots are soft.
2. Put the vegetables in a blender with the water and seasonings. Process until fairly smooth or completely blended, depending on your taste.

Serves 2.

Cool Avocado Soup

1 medium avocado, chopped
2 cups water
2 teaspoons Vogue Vege Base
2 tablespoons dry sherry
1/2 teaspoon sea salt
1/2 teaspoon cumin
1/8 teaspoon cayenne
1/2 small can minced green chiles, drained
1 small sweet* onion, minced

1. Purée avocado in a processor with the water and all the other ingredients except the chiles and onion.
2. Put avocado mixture in a bowl and stir in the chiles and onion. Chill.

*If an onion is too "hot" and not sweet, soak slices in ice water for 15 to 20 minutes, then drain and proceed with recipe.

Serves 2.

Puréed Carrot Soup

1 large, sweet onion, peeled and chopped
2 tablespoons oil
10 carrots, scrubbed and chopped
1 teaspoon freshly grated ginger
2 teaspoons Vogue Vege Base
1/2 cup dry white wine
4 1/2 cups water
1/2 teaspoon allspice
1/2 teaspoon sea salt
1/4 cup minced parsley

1. In a soup pot, sauté onion in oil for 5 minutes. Stir in Vege Base and wine.
2. Add carrots, ginger, water, allspice, and salt and bring to a boil.
3. Lower heat, cover and simmer for 20 minutes or until carrots are soft.
4. Purée in batches in a blender then pour back into the soup pot and reheat.
5. Garnish bowls of soup with parsley.

Serves 4.

NEUTRAL SALADS

The Great American Green Salad

Use fresh, crisp leaf lettuce, romaine, Boston, or any mixed greens. Other optional ingredients: tomato, avocado, celery, carrots, cucumber, mushrooms, scallions, bell peppers, grated beets, broccoli florets, raw turnips, radishes or jicama.

Dressing:
Extra-virgin olive oil and balsamic vinegar in equal parts. Optional: garlic powder and/or Italian seasoning.

For protein meals, you might add toasted pecans, walnuts, sunflower seeds, or cubed soy mozzarella.

For starch meals, garnish with croutons, boiled new potato slices, or beans.

Oriental Salad

2 cups snow peas, strings removed
2 cups small broccoli florets
2 small carrots, thinly sliced
2 cups Chinese cabbage, torn into bite-sized pieces
1 red bell pepper, diced

Dressing:
1/8 cup tamari
1 tablespoon dark sesame oil
1 tablespoon grapeseed oil
1/8 cup brown rice vinegar
1/2 teaspoon minced garlic
1/2 teaspoon fresh grated ginger
2 tablespoons pure water

1. Steam snow peas, broccoli, and carrot for 3 minutes. Rinse in ice water and drain.
2. Combine cabbage and red pepper with the steamed vegetables.
3. Whisk dressing ingredients together and pour over salad. Toss and serve immediately.

Serves 4.

Crunchy Mexican Salad

Use any of the following fresh vegetables, chopped, diced, or sliced. (Everything should be cut small):

Avocado, bell peppers (red or green), carrot, cucumber, celery, jicama, onion, radish, summer squash, and tomato. It's not the same without the avocado and tomato, so include them if possible.

Dressing:
Equal parts umeboshi and white balsamic vinegar. Sea salt, powdered kelp, minced garlic, cayenne, and a small amount of pure water. The amount of each ingredient depends on individual taste, so experiment and make it to suit yours. We like it quite spicy with cayenne.

Put all prepared vegetables in a bowl, whisk together dressing, and pour over vegetables. Toss. Serve immediately.

Southwest Slaw

6 cups shredded green cabbage
1 red bell pepper, diced
1 poblano chili, diced
1 cup jicama, diced
3 scallions, sliced
1/4 cup minced fresh cilantro
Dressing:
Several slices of pickled jalapeños, minced. (To taste)
1/2 teaspoon minced garlic
1/8 cup white balsamic vinegar
1/8 cup olive oil
1/2 teaspoon Herbamare
3 or 4 drops stevia

1. Combine salad ingredients in a large bowl.
2. Whisk together dressing ingredients and stir into salad.
3. Serve or cover and refrigerate.

Serves 6.

NEUTRAL VEGETABLES

Here's a list of the neutral vegetables that I normally use for cooked dishes. Many of them are good simply steamed, baked, or slightly boiled with or without herbs and seasonings. The longer you eat them regularly, the less they seem to need added ingredients: asparagus, beets, broccoli, Brussels sprouts, cabbage, carrots, cauliflower, celery, eggplant, garlic, green beans, greens, leeks, mushrooms, onion, peppers, peas, spinach, wax beans, yellow squash, and zucchini.

If I use tomatoes as a neutral or in a starch dish, I stir them in after the cooking is done.

The secret to delicious and nutritious steamed vegetables is not to overcook them! I steam broccoli only 3 minutes and green beans between 4 and 5. Keep them bright in color and tender-crisp.

If you add an acid-protein such as nuts, tofu, or apple cider vinegar to them while cooking, they are no longer neutral. Likewise, adding flour, oat milk or bread crumbs turns them into alkaline-starch dishes.

Dilled Baby Beets

2 cups of water
12 small spring beets, trimmed, leaving 1/4 inch of leaf tops and roots
    intact to prevent bleeding.
1 tablespoon olive oil
1/2 large, sweet onion, diced
1/2 teaspoon sea salt
2 tablespoons minced, fresh dill

1. In a large saucepan, combine beets and water. Bring to a boil, cover, lower heat and simmer for about 20 minutes, or until beets are tender.
2. Meanwhile, in a large skillet, heat oil and sauté onion until it is translucent. Remove from heat and stir in the salt and dill.
3. When beets are done, trim off stems and roots, cut in halves and combine with the onion-dill mixture. Heat lightly, tossing to coat the beets.

Serves 4.

Four Color Stir-Fry

1 tablespoon grapeseed oil
2 medium carrots, sliced
1/4 head of small cauliflower florets
16 snow peas, trimmed
1 red bell pepper, cut in strips

1. In a wok or skillet, heat oil. Add carrots and a small amount of water. Cover and steam for 4 minutes.
2. Add broccoli, cover, and steam for 3 minutes. Remove cover.
3. Add snow peas and bell pepper. Stir-fry on high heat for 1 to 2 minutes.

Serves 4.

Stir-fried Kale with Garlic

Art swore that he hated kale until I prepared this dish. We were both pleased at how sweet and delicious it was.

1 bunch kale (or collard greens)
4 cups water
1 tablespoon grapeseed oil
1 teaspoon minced garlic

1. Wash and trim leaves by cutting out the stems. Stack leaves, 4 at a time and cut into thin strips.
2. In a large saucepan, bring water to a boil and submerge kale. Cover, bring back to a boil, lower heat and simmer for 5 minutes. Drain kale.
3. In a skillet, heat oil and garlic. Add kale and stir-fry for just a minute or 2, until heated and well mixed.

(Optional, season with salt and/or a little white balsamic vinegar)

Serves 2 to 4.

Balsamic Glazed Onions

2 large, sweet onions, thinly sliced
1 tablespoon grapeseed oil
1/4 cup balsamic vinegar

1. Heat oil in a large skillet.
2. Add onions and sauté for 12 minutes. Add vinegar and simmer, stirring, until the vinegar has nearly evaporated.

Serves 4.

Puréed Vegetables with Roasted Garlic

1 head of garlic
1/2 teaspoon olive oil
4 cups of water
1 teaspoon salt
1 rutabaga, peeled and chopped
3 carrots, scrubbed and chopped
2 parsnips, scrubbed and chopped
1 teaspoon dried rosemary
1/2 teaspoon Herbamare
2 tablespoons grapeseed oil

1. Heat oven to 400 degrees.
2. Cut off top of garlic, exposing the cloves, and drizzle with olive oil. Wrap in foil and bake for 45 minutes.
3. Meanwhile, in a large pot, combine water and salt and bring to a boil.
4. Put the vegetables in, cover and bring back to a boil. Lower heat and simmer until vegetables are soft. Drain.
5. In a processor, in batches, purée vegetables and squeezed-out garlic cloves with the rosemary, Herbamare, and oil. Process until smooth and stir it all together to mix well.
6. Garnish each serving with paprika.

Serves 6.

Carrots with Coriander

1 tablespoon grapeseed oil
1/2 large, sweet onion, diced
4 carrots, sliced
1 teaspoon ground coriander
1/2 teaspoon Herbamare
2 teaspoons white balsamic vinegar
1/3 cup water
1 tablespoon fresh, minced parsley

1. In a saucepan, heat oil and sauté onion for 5 minutes.
2. Add all other ingredients except the parsley. Cover, bring to a boil, lower heat and simmer until carrots are just tender, not soft.
3. Drain and serve garnished with parsley.

Serves 4.

Roasted Vegetables

4 small yellow squash, cut into 1-inch slices
4 small zucchini, cut into 1-inch slices
2 onions, quartered
2 tablespoons olive oil
2 teaspoons oregano
1/2 teaspoon Herbamare
dash of cayenne
2 large red bell peppers, cut into 1/2-inch strips
2 green bell peppers, cut into 1/2-inch strips
2 tablespoons balsamic vinegar
1/4 cup chopped parsley

1. Heat oven to 500 degrees.
2. Toss squash and onions in oil, oregano, and Herbamare. Place in a baking pan and roast for 10 minutes.
3. Add pepper strips. Roast 10 more minutes, until they begin to char.
4. Transfer to a bowl. Add vinegar and parsley. Toss gently.

Serves 4.

Garlic Green Beans or Broccoli

1 pound of trimmed green beans or two bunches of small broccoli
florets, steamed
1 tablespoon olive oil
2 teaspoons minced garlic
1/2 teaspoon lemon-pepper
1/4 teaspoon Spike all-purpose seasoning
1/3 cup minced fresh parsley

1. Cook beans in boiling water for 5 minutes, or steam broccoli for 3 minutes.
2. In a large skillet, heat oil and sauté garlic.
3. Add seasonings then add beans or broccoli and stir-fry for 2 minutes. Spoon into serving dish.

Serves 4 to 6.

Baked Carrots and Onions

1 large, sweet onion, cut in quarters
4 carrots, cut in half, then halved lengthwise
1/2 cup pure water
1 tablespoon tamari
1 tablespoon grapeseed oil
1/2 teaspoon tarragon

1. Heat oven to 375 degrees.
2. Oil a baking dish with a lid and arrange onions and carrots in the dish.
3. Whisk water, tamari, oil, and tarragon together and pour over the vegetables.
4. Cover and bake for 45 minutes, basting occasionally with the broth.

Serves 4.

Carrots, Zucchini and Peas

2 medium carrots, grated
2 zucchini, grated
1 large, sweet onion, diced
1 tablespoon grapeseed oil
1 teaspoon minced garlic
1/8 cup dry white wine
1 package frozen peas
1 tablespoon tamari

1. Heat oil in a skillet and sauté onion for 5 minutes. Add garlic, carrots, zucchini, and wine. Cover and simmer for 5 minutes.
2. Meanwhile, put frozen peas in a colander and run very hot water over them until they are completely thawed.
3. Remove lid from skillet. Add peas and sprinkle the tamari over all. Raise the heat and cook, stirring until all the liquid is gone. Serve immediately.

Serves 4.

Steamed Cabbage

1/2 green cabbage, cut in wedges
2 tablespoons roasted sesame seeds

1. Put water in a steaming pot, bring to a boil. Place cabbage in steamer. Steam for 4 minutes.
2. Remove cabbage from steamer and sprinkle on sesame seeds.

Serves 4.

NEUTRAL SAUCES

Red Bell Pepper Sauce

2 large bell peppers
1/4 teaspoon salt
1/2 teaspoon minced garlic
1 teaspoon balsamic vinegar

1. Core peppers and cut into large chunks. Steam for 10 to 15 minutes, until very soft.
2. Put peppers and other ingredients in a food processor and purée until smooth.
3. Strain through a sieve into a bowl.
4. Serve at room temperature on omelets, vegetables or grains.

Mushroom Sauce

2 teaspoons grapeseed oil
1/2 onion, diced
1/2 teaspoon salt
1 teaspoon minced garlic
8 mushrooms, finely chopped
1/2 cup water
1/8 cup red wine
1 tablespoon tamari

1. In a skillet, heat oil, put in onions, and sprinkle with the salt. Sauté until onion is golden. Add mushrooms and cover. Simmer for 5 minutes.
2. Add the rest of the ingredients and cook, covered for 15 more minutes.

Quick Brown Sauce

1 tablespoon instant minced onion
1 teaspoon minced garlic
2 teaspoons tekka
1 tablespoon oil
1 teaspoon Vogue Vege Base
1 cup water
2 tablespoons tamari
1/2 cup red wine
2 teaspoons kudzu dissolved in 2 tablespoons water

1. Sauté onion, garlic, and tekka in the oil for 2 minutes.
2. Stir in the rest of the ingredients except kudzu and simmer for 5 minutes.
3. Add dissolved kudzu and simmer, stirring until smooth and thickened.

White Wine Sauce

1 tablespoon olive oil
1/2 teaspoon minced garlic
2 cloves
1/4 teaspoon thyme
1/8 teaspoon tarragon
1 tablespoon minced parsley
1 cup dry white wine
2 teaspoons drained capers (optional)
2 teaspoons arrowroot dissolved in 1 tablespoon water

1. Heat oil in a saucepan and sauté garlic for 1 minute.
2. Add the rest of the ingredients except the capers and arrowroot and simmer for 10 minutes.
3. Remove the cloves. Stir in the dissolved arrowroot and capers, if using, and simmer until thickened.

Good on fish or vegetables.

Shiitaki Gravy

4 dried shiitake mushrooms, stems removed and soaked in 1 1/4
    cups <u>hot</u> water for 30 minutes
1 tablespoon grapeseed oil
1/2 onion, diced
1 teaspoon minced garlic
1/2 teaspoon oregano
1 1/2 tablespoons Bragg's amino acids
1/8 cup red wine
1 tablespoon arrowroot dissolved in 2 tablespoons water

1. Sauté onion in oil until it turns a golden brown. Add garlic and oregano and cook another minute.
2. Chop mushrooms and add to the onion mixture. Pour in the mushroom soaking water, leaving any sediment out.
3. Stir in the amino acids and the wine, cover and simmer 35 minutes. Add salt if needed, to taste.
4. Stir in dissolved arrowroot and simmer until thick. Good on tofu or tempeh.

ALKALINE-STARCH APPETIZERS

Lentil Paté

2 teaspoons olive oil
1 small onion, diced
1 cup brown lentils
1 cup water
1/2 cup white wine
1/2 avocado, peeled and chopped
2 tablespoons lemon juice
1/4 teaspoon salt
dash of kelp and cayenne

1. In a large saucepan, sauté onion in oil for 5 minutes.
2. Stir in water and lentils, bring to a boil, lower heat, cover, and simmer until lentils are tender, about 40 minutes.
3. Drain lentil mixture, reserving the juice, and purée in a processor, adding the reserved juice as necessary to make a smooth paste.
4. Add avocado, lemon juice, and seasonings and process again until very smooth.
5. Spoon into a bowl, cover and chill for several hours.

Good on crisp breads or crackers.

Aduki Bean Dip

1 cup aduki beans
3 cups water
1 strip kombu
2 tablespoons grapeseed oil
1 1/2 tablespoons freshly grated ginger
1 tablespoon balsamic vinegar
1/8 teaspoon cayenne
sea salt to taste

1. In a large saucepan, combine beans, water, and kombu. Bring to a boil, lower heat, cover, and simmer for 1 1/2 hours. Remove kombu and drain beans, reserving water.
2. Purée beans and a little of the water adding the rest of the ingredients until it is a smooth dip consistency.

Carrot Paté

1 tablespoon olive oil
1 small onion, chopped
3 carrots, chopped
1/4 cup water
1/4 cup orange juice
1 tablespoon grated orange zest
1/2 teaspoon salt
1/8 teaspoon curry powder
1/2 small avocado
1 tablespoon white balsamic vinegar

1. In a large saucepan, sauté onion in oil for 5 minutes.
2. Add carrots, water, orange juice, orange zest, salt, and curry powder. Bring to a boil, lower heat, cover and simmer for 5 to 10 minutes, until the liquid has evaporated.
3. In a processor, purée carrot mixture until smooth. Add avocado and vinegar and process until well combined.
4. Spoon paté into a small bowl, cover, and chill for several hours.

White Bean Paté

1/3 cup chopped onion
1 teaspoon minced garlic
2 cans white beans, rinsed and drained
1 tablespoon capers
1 tablespoon white balsamic vinegar
1 tablespoon olive oil
1/2 teaspoon each: dried basil, thyme, dill, and tarragon
1/2 teaspoon sea salt, or to taste
1/8 teaspoon cayenne
1/4 teaspoon coriander
1/4 cup fresh, minced parsley

1. In a processor, purée onion and garlic.
2. Add beans and all other ingredients except the parsley and process until smooth.
3. Stir in parsley, adjust seasonings.

Good on crisp breads and crackers and also makes a good sandwich filling.

Red Bell Pepper Dip

6 red bell peppers, roasted and peeled (or a large jar of prepared roasted peppers)
3 tablespoons olive oil
3 tablespoons balsamic vinegar
1 teaspoon ground cumin
1/4 teaspoon cayenne
1 teaspoon honey

In a processor, purée all ingredients until smooth.
Serve with raw or steamed vegetables or triangles of pita bread.
Also good as a sandwich spread.

Mushroom Crostini

1 1/2 teaspoons minced garlic
1 tablespoon olive oil
1 pound button mushrooms, thinly sliced
1/3 cup dry sherry
Thin strips of roasted bell pepper
1 loaf of whole grain, crusty bread cut in 1/2" thick slices
1/4 cup minced parsley

1. In a large skillet, sauté garlic in oil for 1 minute. Add mushrooms and sherry and cook for about 10 minutes or until liquid has evaporated, stirring occasionally.
2. Heat broiler and toast bread.
3. Top each bread slice with mushroom mixture and a strip of bell pepper and sprinkle with parsley.

Roasted Garbanzo Beans

2 cans organic garbanzo beans, rinsed and drained. Place on paper towels to dry
1/8 cup olive oil
1/2 teaspoon each: salt, cumin, and coriander
1/4 teaspoon cayenne

1. Heat oven to 400 degrees.
2. Toss beans with oil and seasonings.
3. Spread beans on a non-stick baking sheet and bake for 35 to 45 minutes, shaking the pan occasionally, until they are golden brown and crisp.

Eat like popcorn.

Roasted Sweet Onion and Garlic Spread

2 large sweet onions (Texas 1015's, Maui, Walla Walla Sweets, Vidalia, or other)
2 teaspoons olive oil
2 teaspoons honey
6 garlic cloves, peeled
1/4 teaspoon salt

1. Heat oven to 350 degrees.
2. Peel and quarter onions.
3. In a large bowl, combine oil Add onions and garlic, stirring to coat.
4. Transfer to an oiled baking dish and bake, uncovered, for 40 minutes, stirring occasionally.
5. Cool slightly and transfer to a processor. Add salt and purée until very smooth. Add honey.

Good on whole grain, crusty bread or crackers. Also good as a sandwich spread. Keeps up to a week, covered, in the refrigerator.

Baked Garlic on Toast

Baked garlic, by itself is neutral; however, you can use it to spread on toast, crusty bread, or crackers in place of butter.
2 heads of garlic
2 teaspoons of olive oil

1. Heat oven to 350 degrees.
2. Slice top off of garlic heads revealing cloves. Sprinkle tops with oil.
3. Wrap in foil or place in a garlic baker.
4. Bake for 45 minutes, or until cloves easily squeeze out of peel.

Serves 4 as an appetizer or use it as a substitute for butter with your meal on baked potatoes, or ears of corn, etc.

STARCH - ALKALINE SOUPS

Baked Potato Soup

2 large baking potatoes, scrubbed
1 head garlic
1 tablespoon oil
1 small onion, diced
1 teaspoon oil
1 tablespoon Vogue Vege Base
2 1/2 cups water
1 teaspoon Herbamare
1/2 teaspoon dill
dash of cayenne

1. Heat oven to 350 degrees.
2. Pierce potatoes with a fork and cut the top off the head of garlic to expose the cloves. Drizzle olive oil over the top of the garlic and wrap in foil.
3. Place potatoes and garlic in the oven and bake for 1 hour. Remove garlic. Bake potatoes another 30 minutes.
4. In a medium saucepan, sauté the onion in oil for 10 minutes.
5. Add the water, Herbamare, dill and cayenne to the onion. Squeeze garlic cloves out of the head and into the pan. (They should slip out easily).
6. Just before potatoes are done, bring the mixture to a boil.
7. Chop 1 potato, including skin and put in a blender along with the water mixture. Blend until smooth. Pour back into the pan.
8. Chop the second potato including skin in small pieces and stir it into the soup mixture.

Serves 2 as a main dish with a salad.
Serves 4 as a first course.

Lima Bean Soup

2 cups large, dry lima beans
1 strip kombu
1 tablespoon olive oil
1 large onion, minced
2 carrots, minced
2 teaspoons thyme
1/2 teaspoon kelp powder
dash cayenne
sea salt to taste

1. Soak beans overnight in water to cover, plus about 6 inches.
2. Drain off soaking water. Cover beans with fresh water to cover, plus about 2 inches. Tuck kombu under the beans.
3. Bring beans to a boil. Lower heat, cover and simmer for about an hour (until beans are soft).
4. Meanwhile, sauté onion, carrot, kelp and thyme in the oil for 20 minutes.
5. Remove kombu from the beans. Purée half of the beans and cooking liquid in a blender. Pour back into beans.
6. Stir onion, carrot mixture into the beans and season to taste.

Serves 4.

Lentil Soup

2 tablespoons olive oil
1 large onion, diced
4 stalks celery, diced
2 carrots, diced
2 teaspoons minced garlic
4 cups water
1 cup brown lentils
2 tablespoons tamari
1 tablespoon dried parsley
1 teaspoon sea salt
1/2 teaspoon each: dried basil, thyme and oregano
1/8 teaspoon each: cayenne and kelp

1. In a large saucepan, sauté vegetables in oil for 5 minutes.
2. Add water and lentils, bring to a boil lower heat, cover and simmer 1 hour.
3. Add the rest of ingredients and simmer another 10 minutes, stir frequently.

Serves 4.

"Healing" Vegetable Soup

This is a great soup to keep on hand. Use organic vegetables whenever possible. It keeps in the refrigerator for several days. Use different vegetables according to your taste, but don't leave out the cabbage and the kale.

1 tablespoon olive oil
1 large yellow onion, diced
2 stalks celery, diced
4 carrots, sliced
1/2 small head cabbage, sliced into small shreds
3 leaves of kale, stems trimmed off and leaves sliced as cabbage
2 large potatoes, scrubbed and diced
1/4 pound fresh green beans, trimmed and cut into 1-inch pieces
2 zucchini, sliced
4 small yellow squash, sliced
3 tablespoons Vogue Vege Base
2 quarts of water
1 1/2 tablespoons fines herbs
Dash of cayenne and kelp
Sea salt to taste

1. In a large soup pot, sauté onion, celery and carrots in oil for 5 minutes.
2. Stir in Vege Base, water and all other vegetables except the squash. Bring to a boil, lower heat, cover and simmer for 45 minutes.
3. Add squash, fines herbs, cayenne and kelp and simmer another 15 minutes.
4. Season to taste.

Serves 4.

Variations:
1. Add a can of organic navy beans or puréed beans along with the squash.
2. Instead of fines herbs, use an Italian seasoning blend.
3. With Italian seasoning, add cooked pasta before serving.

Split Pea Soup

1 tablespoon olive oil
1 medium onion, diced
1 carrot, scrubbed and chopped
1 stalk celery, diced
4 cups water
1 cup split peas
1/2 teaspoon each: marjoram, thyme, basil, celery seed, and sea salt
1/4 teaspoon kelp
1 bay leaf
1/4 cup parsley, minced

1. In a large saucepan, sauté onion, carrot, and celery for 10 minutes.
2. Add water, split peas, and bay leaf. Bring to a boil, lower heat, cover and simmer for 30 minutes.
3. Add the herbs and seasonings and simmer another 15 minutes.
4. Remove bay leaf. Purée in a blender leaving bits of carrot intact.
5. Garnish with parsley.

Serves 2.

Golden Bisque

1 tablespoon olive oil
1 medium onion, chopped
2 carrots, chopped
1 small butternut squash, peeled, seeded and chopped
1/2 head of cauliflower florets
2 tablespoons Vogue Vege Base
6 cups water (more, if needed, to cover vegetables)
1/2 cup rolled oats
2 teaspoons sea salt
1/2 teaspoon kelp
1 teaspoon dill
dash cayenne

1. In a large soup pot, sauté onion and carrot in the oil for 10 minutes.
2. Add the Vege Base, water, squash, cauliflower, oats, and seasonings. Bring to a boil, lower heat, cover and simmer for 45 minutes.
3. Purée in a blender in batches.

Serves 4.

Quick Black Bean Soup

2 15-ounce cans organic black beans
1 tablespoon dried onion flakes
1 teaspoon minced garlic
1 teaspoon cumin
1 teaspoon Herbamare
Dash of cayenne
1 1/4 cups water
3/4 cup orange juice

1. Put beans in a colander and rinse under hot water.
2. Blend half of the beans with the rest of the ingredients. Pour into a saucepan. Stir in remaining beans, heat and serve.

Serves 4.

Quick Cream of Celery Soup

5 stalks of celery, trimmed and chopped
1/2 onion, diced
1 large potato, scrubbed and diced
1 cup of water
2 cups of oat milk
1 1/2 teaspoon dried parsley
1 teaspoon basil
1 teaspoon Herbamare
2 teaspoons Vogue Vege Base

1. Combine all ingredients in a large saucepan. Bring to a boil, lower heat, cover and simmer for 20 minutes.
2. Blend in batches until smooth.

Serves 2.

ALKALINE-STARCH SALADS

Complete Meal Quinoa Salad

Quinoa is one of my favorite grains. It cooks quickly and adapts itself to a great many dishes. Always rinse the grains well (in a sieve) before cooking.

1 cup rinsed quinoa
2 cups pure water
1/2 teaspoon salt
2 cups small broccoli florets, steamed for 3 minutes.
2 zucchini, diced
1 1/2 cups diced fennel bulb
1 red bell pepper, diced
1/2 cup oil-packed, sun-dried tomatoes, minced.
1/4 cup capers, drained
1 can organic black beans, rinsed and drained

Dressing:
1/4 cup olive oil
1/4 cup brown rice vinegar
1/8 cup balsamic vinegar
1 teaspoon Herbamare

1. Combine water, salt, and quinoa in a medium saucepan. Bring to a boil, lower heat, cover and simmer for 15 minutes.
2. Meanwhile, prepare the vegetables.
3. Cool the quinoa and combine with the vegetables.
4. Whisk dressing ingredients together and pour over quinoa mixture, tossing gently to combine.

Can be served at room temperature or kept in the refrigerator. Covered, it will keep in the refrigerator for several days.

Serves 6.

Quinoa Stir-Fried Vegetable Salad

1 cup rinsed quinoa
2 cups pure water
1 tablespoon Vogue Vege Base
1/2 teaspoon salt
2 tablespoons olive oil
2 teaspoons minced garlic
1 large sweet onion, diced
2 stalks celery, diced
10 snow peas, trimmed and cut in thirds
2 zucchini, diced
1/2 teaspoon marjoram, crushed
2 roasted red bell peppers, chopped
2 large ripe tomatoes, chopped
1/4 cup umeboshi vinegar
1/4 cup sesame oil

1. Combine quinoa, water, Vege Base, and salt in a medium saucepan. Bring to a boil, lower heat, cover and simmer for 15 minutes.
2. Meanwhile, in a large skillet or wok, sauté garlic, onions, and celery in the oil for 2 minutes.
3. Add snow peas, zucchini, and marjoram and cook, stirring, about 2 more minutes, until vegetables are crisp, tender.
4. Combine quinoa, cooked vegetables, peppers, and tomatoes. Sprinkle vinegar and oil over all, mixing and seasoning to taste.

Serves 6.

Garbanzo Salad

1 sweet onion, diced
1 15-ounce can garbanzo beans, rinsed and drained
1 ripe tomato, diced
1 green bell pepper, diced
1/4 cup minced fresh parsley
2 tablespoons umeboshi vinegar
1/4 cup white balsamic vinegar
1/8 cup olive oil
2 teaspoons minced garlic
salt and cayenne to taste

1. Combine first 5 ingredients in a bowl.
2. Whisk the rest of the ingredients together and mix with beans. Let marinate overnight.

Serves 2.

Black-Eyed Pea-Sweet Potato Salad

2 large sweet potatoes, baked and peeled
2 16-ounce cans black-eyed peas, rinsed and drained
1 package frozen corn (thawed completely by immersing in boiling
     water for a few minutes)
1/8 cup fresh parsley, minced
4 scallions, sliced

Dressing:
3 tablespoons balsamic vinegar
3 tablespoons brown rice vinegar
3 tablespoons olive oil
1 teaspoon Dijon mustard
1/2 teaspoon sea salt
dash of cayenne and kelp

1. Chop potatoes, combine with vegetables.
2. Whisk dressing ingredients together, toss with vegetables.
Serves 6.

Southwest Lentil Salad

1 1/2 cups brown lentils
6 cups water
12 ripe cherry tomatoes, quartered
1 carrot, diced
1 stalk celery, diced
1/2 large sweet onion, diced
1/3 cup finely minced parsley
Dressing:
2 to 4 pickled jalapeño slices, minced
1/2 teaspoon Tabasco
1/2 teaspoon minced garlic
1/4 cup balsamic vinegar
1/8 cup brown rice vinegar
1/8 cup olive oil
Herbamare to taste

1. In a saucepan, combine lentils and water. Bring to a boil, lower heat, cover and simmer for about 25 minutes, until lentils are tender but not soft.
2. Drain lentils in a colander. Run cold water over the lentils and drain well.
3. Combine lentils with vegetables.
4. Whisk together the dressing ingredients and season to taste (it should be highly seasoned). Pour over salad, tossing gently to mix.
5. Serve at room temperature.

Serves 6.

Texas Caviar

1 can black-eyed peas, rinsed and drained
1 sweet onion, peeled and diced
1 green bell pepper, diced
1 red bell pepper, diced
2 stalks celery, diced
1 carrot, scrubbed and diced
2 tablespoons capers, drained
6 pickled jalapeño slices, drained and minced
1/8 cup olive oil
1/8 cup balsamic vinegar
1/2 teaspoon sea salt

1. Combine first 7 ingredients in a large bowl.
2. Whisk together the jalapeño, olive oil, salt, and vinegar. Pour over the vegetables and toss lightly to mix well.
3. Cover and refrigerate at least 2 hours to let flavors blend.

Serves 4.

Taco Salad

1 bunch leaf lettuce, washed, dried, and torn into bite-size pieces
1 large tomato, chopped
1 avocado, chopped
1/4 cup sliced ripe olives
2 scallions, sliced
1/3 green bell pepper, diced
1/8 cup minced cilantro
3 cups baked tortilla chips

Dressing:
1/8 cup olive oil
2 tablespoons white balsamic vinegar
1 tablespoon umeboshi vinegar
1/2 teaspoon each: sea salt and garlic
1/4 teaspoon each: cayenne and chili powder

1. Whisk together all dressing ingredients and toss with vegetables.
2. Arrange on salad plates and garnish with baked tortilla chips.

Serves 4.

Spanish Rice Salad

1 cup Texmati brown rice
2 cups pure water
1/2 teaspoon sea salt
3 ripe tomatoes, chopped
2 stalks celery, diced
1/4 cup sliced, stuffed olives
2 zucchini, diced

Dressing:
1/2 onion, chopped
1/4 cup grapeseed oil
1/4 cup brown rice vinegar
1/8 cup balsamic vinegar
1 teaspoon cumin
1/4 teaspoon cayenne
1 teaspoon minced garlic
1/4 cup water

1. Put rice, water, and salt in a saucepan, bring to a boil, lower heat, cover and simmer for 50 minutes. Do not lift lid and do not stir.
2. In a blender, combine all dressing ingredients and blend until smooth.
3. Pour dressing into a small saucepan and bring to a simmer. Cook for 10 minutes.
4. When rice is done, combine with the vegetables and pour on the hot dressing. Mix well.
5. Serve at room temperature or cover and refrigerate.

Serves 4.

White Bean-Horseradish Salad

2 15-ounce cans organic navy beans
1 carrot, diced
1 stalk celery, diced
1 red bell pepper, diced
1/2 cup pitted, chopped green olives

Dressing:
1/4 cup olive oil
1/8 cup white balsamic vinegar
1/8 cup brown rice vinegar
1/4 cup prepared horseradish
1 teaspoon dried rosemary, crushed
1/2 teaspoon Herbamare
1/4 teaspoon cayenne

Whisk together dressing ingredients and pour over vegetables.
Toss well. Let sit an hour before serving.

Serves 4.

Chinese Quinoa Salad

1 cup rinsed quinoa
2 cups pure water
1/2 teaspoon sea salt
1 carrot, scrubbed and diced
2 cups small broccoli florets
1 large cucumber, peeled, seeded and diced
4 scallions, finely sliced
2 celery stalks, diced

Dressing:
1/8 cup grapeseed oil
2 tablespoons roasted sesame oil
1/8 cup tamari
2 tablespoons brown rice vinegar
1 tablespoon ume vinegar
2 teaspoons freshly grated ginger
1/4 cup roasted sesame seeds*

1. Put quinoa, water, and salt in a medium saucepan, bring to a boil, lower heat, cover and simmer for 15 minutes.
2. Meanwhile, steam the diced carrot and broccoli for 3 minutes.
3. Whisk together all the dressing ingredients.
4. When the quinoa is cooked, combine with all the vegetables and stir in the dressing.
5. Cover and refrigerate for an hour or so to let the flavors develop.

Serves 4.

*To roast sesame seeds, spread out in a skillet and heat, stirring until they are golden tan and the aroma rises. Be careful not to burn.

SANDWICHES

There are so many possibilities for really delicious sandwiches that I will only try to get you started. Creating your own specialties is part of the fun.

Select good whole-grain breads, flat breads, tortillas, or pitas and select your favorite fillings from the list below.

Just remember that the nature of a sandwich starts with a starch, so any filling has to be neutral or a starch.

Avocado	Mushroom	Tomato
Cucumber	Grated carrot	Lettuce
Sprouts	Onion	Olive
Bean spread	Peppers	Radish
Watercress	Grilled veggies	

Use any spread you like, mustard, mayo, or whatever. The little bit of acid or protein in the spread will not hurt.

One of my favorite sandwiches is a grilled portabella mushroom drizzled with balsamic vinegar.

ALKALINE-STARCH VEGETABLES

Butternut Squash-Orange Purée

1 medium butternut squash
1 large orange, grated rind and juiced

1. Heat oven to 375 degrees.
2. Cut squash in half. Remove seeds. Place cut side down in a baking dish. Bake for 45 minutes, or until tender.
3. In the meantime, grate orange rind and extract juice. When the squash is done, spoon meat out and put into a processor. Add orange juice and rind.
4. Add salt to taste and (optional) a dash of coriander or nutmeg.
5. Purée until smooth.

Serves 4.

Pineapple-Glazed Carrots

4 medium carrots, sliced
1/2 cup pineapple juice
1/2 teaspoon cinnamon
1/8 teaspoon nutmeg
dash cayenne

Combine all ingredients in a saucepan. Simmer 10 minutes. Serve hot. Salt to taste.

Serves 4.

Braised Red Cabbage

1 tablespoon olive oil
1 large, sweet onion, thinly sliced
1/2 teaspoon Herbamare
1 small red cabbage, thinly shredded
1 small apple, cored and diced
1/8 cup balsamic vinegar
1/3 cup water
1/3 cup apple juice

1. Heat oven to 375 degrees.
2. Heat oil in a skillet and add the onion and Herbamare. Sauté for 5 minutes.
3. Add the cabbage and apple and cook for another 5 minutes. (Add small amount of water if needed to prevent sticking.)
4. Combine the vinegar, water, and apple juice and pour over the cabbage, mixing well.
5. Oil a baking dish with cover, and spoon cabbage and liquid into dish. Cover and bake for 45 minutes.

Serves 6.

Sweet Fall Squash Medley

1 buttercup squash, peeled, seeded and chopped
2 sweet potatoes, peeled and chopped
1/8 cup grapeseed oil
2 tablespoons honey
1 tablespoon grated orange rind
1/4 cup orange juice
1/2 teaspoon cinnamon
1/4 teaspoon nutmeg
2 small, tart apples, peeled, cored, and sliced

1. Heat oven to 350 degrees.
2. Oil a baking dish and arrange squash and sweet potatoes in it. Set aside.
3. Combine oil and next 5 ingredients in a small saucepan. Bring to a boil, stirring constantly, then pour over the squash-potato mixture.
4. Cover. Bake for 30 minutes. Uncover and stir in apple. Bake for another 30 minutes, uncovered.

Serves 6.

Acorn Squash Purée

2 acorn squash
1 tablespoon olive oil
1 tablespoon maple syrup
1/2 teaspoon salt
1/2 teaspoon allspice

1. Heat oven to 375 degrees.
2. Oil baking dish. Halve and seed squash. Place cut side down in dish and add water to a depth of 1/4 inch.
3. Bake for 45 minutes. Drain and cool slightly.
4. Scoop out pulp, place in a food processor with the other ingredients purée until smooth.
5. Add salt if needed.

Serves 4.

Baked Garlic Potatoes

1 head of garlic
1 teaspoon olive oil
2 large baking potatoes, scrubbed
1/2 cup water
1 teaspoon Vogue Vege Broth
1/2 teaspoon salt
dash cayenne

1. Heat oven to 425 degrees.
2. Cut top off of garlic to expose cloves. Drizzle with oil. Wrap in foil.
3. Pierce potatoes. Put potatoes and garlic in the oven. Bake 45 minutes.
4. Remove garlic from oven. Continue baking potato another 25 minutes.
5. Halve potatoes lengthwise. Scoop out pulp, reserving shells.
6. Squeeze garlic cloves out into potato pulp. Add next 3 ingredients. Mash until smooth and creamy.
7. Spoon into shells. Bake 10 minutes. Garnish with paprika.

Serves 4.

Scalloped Potatoes

2 large potatoes, peeled and sliced
1 large, sweet onion, peeled and sliced
2 teaspoons of arrowroot dissolved in
2 cups oat milk
2 teaspoons Vogue Vege Base
1 teaspoon Herbamare
1 teaspoon minced garlic
1/4 teaspoon cayenne
salt to taste

1. Heat oven to 375 degrees. Oil a baking dish with a lid.
2. Layer potatoes and onions in the dish.
3. Combine the rest of the ingredients and pour over the potatoes. Sprinkle top with paprika if desired.
4. Cover and bake for 45 minutes. Remove lid and continue baking until golden brown.

Serves 4.

Stuffed Squash

4 small acorn squash
1 1/2 cup pure water
2 teaspoons Vogue Vege Base
1/2 cup raisins
1 tablespoon olive oil
1 large onion, minced
3 stalks celery, minced
2 teaspoons minced garlic
2 Fuji or Gala apples, cored and diced
1 1/2 cups whole grain bread finely diced
2 tablespoons minced flat-leaf parsley
2 tablespoons fresh minced thyme or basil
2 teaspoons lemon zest
1/2 teaspoon Herbamare

1. Heat oven to 350 degrees. Oil baking dish.
2. Cut squash in halves from top to bottom. Trim top and bottom so they sit flat. Scoop out seeds. Bake cut side down for 40 minutes. Remove from oven and cool.
3. Meanwhile, heat water and Vege Base to boiling. Pour into raisins and set aside.
4. Heat oil in a large skillet. Sauté onion, celery and garlic until soft. Add the apple and cook for about 2 minutes. Remove from heat and stir in bread, herbs, lemon zest, drained raisins (reserve the liquid) and Herbamare.
5. Add the reserved liquid a little at a time, stirring, until the stuffing is moist but not wet. Add more Herbamare to taste, if needed.
6. Spoon stuffing into the baked squash, piling high.
7. Raise oven temperature to 375 and bake for 20 minutes.

Serves 8.

Spiced Mixed "Fries"

1 large baking potato, peeled and sliced
1 large sweet potato, peeled and sliced
1 medium turnip, peeled and sliced
1/8 cup grapeseed oil
1 teaspoon each: chili powder, garlic powder and Herbamare

1. Heat oven to 350 degrees.
2. Combine oil and seasonings. Toss with vegetables to coat.
3. Spread vegetables out on 2 baking trays and bake for 30 to 40 minutes. (Try one to make sure they are done.)
4. Place under broiler for a few minutes just before serving, but watch carefully to see that they are just a golden brown.

Serves 4.

Sherried Sweet Potatoes

4 large sweet potatoes
1/8 cup dry sherry
1/4 cup maple syrup
1/2 teaspoon ground ginger
1/2 teaspoon nutmeg
sea salt to taste

1. Heat oven to 375 degrees.
2. Bake sweet potatoes for 1 1/2 hours. Cool and peel and mash with a potato masher.
3. Mix sherry, maple syrup, and seasonings together then stir into the potatoes. Salt to taste.
4. Spread potatoes evenly in an oiled pan and bake at 375 degrees for about 15 minutes, until hot.

Serves 8.

ALKALINE-STARCH SAUCES

Brown Mushroom Sauce

4 dried shiitake mushrooms, stems removed
1 cup boiling water
6 button mushrooms, chopped
1 tablespoon olive oil
1/2 teaspoon minced garlic
2 teaspoons tekka
1/4 cup dry sherry
1 tablespoon tamari
2 teaspoons kudzu dissolved in 1 tablespoon water

1. Soak the shiitake mushrooms for 30 minutes. Remove from soaking water (reserve water) and squeeze lightly. Slice into thin strips.
2. Heat the oil and sauté all the mushrooms for 10 minutes. Stir in the garlic, tekka, sherry, and the soaking water (strain out the sediment). Simmer 5 more minutes.
3. Add the soy sauce and dissolved kuzu and simmer, stirring until smooth and thickened.

This sauce is great on grains or baked potatoes.

Stir-Fry Sauce

1/3 cup orange juice
1/8 cup tamari
1 tablespoon grated ginger
1 teaspoon minced garlic
1 tablespoon honey
2 teaspoons sesame oil
2 teaspoons kudzu dissolved in 1 tablespoon water

1. Whisk together the first 6 ingredients then stir in the dissolved kudzu.
2. Stir into stir-fried vegetables just before they are finished cooking. Simmer a few seconds and toss to coat vegetables well.

Beautiful Beet Sauce

2 medium-sized beets
1 1/2 cups water
1/2 cup orange juice
2 tablespoons balsamic vinegar
1 teaspoon honey
1/2 teaspoon salt

1. In a small saucepan, cook beets in water until soft. (About 30 minutes)
2. Remove beets from water and let cool enough to handle. Rub off skins.
3. In a blender, purée beets with the orange juice, vinegar, honey, and salt.

To serve, pour a puddle of the sauce on the plate and lay a vegetable or a vegetable medley, on top.

Orange-Ginger Sauce

1 teaspoon grated orange rind
1 cup orange juice
1 teaspoon minced garlic
1 tablespoon grated ginger
1/8 cup tamari
1/8 cup dry sherry
1 scallion, finely sliced
2 teaspoons kudzu dissolved in 2 teaspoons water

1. In a saucepan, combine orange rind, orange juice, garlic, ginger, tamari and sherry. Bring to a boil,
2. Stir in the dissolved kudzu and cook, stirring, until thickened.

This is good on stir-fried vegetables, grains, or a flat bread filled like a crepe with steamed vegetables and topped with this sauce.

Sweet and Sour Sauce

1 cup apple juice
1 teaspoon honey
2 tablespoons cider vinegar
2 teaspoons grated ginger
1 teaspoon minced garlic
1/2 cup small pineapple chunks
2 teaspoons kudzu dissolved in 2 teaspoons water

1. In a saucepan, combine first 6 ingredients and bring to a boil.
2. Lower heat and stir in the dissolved kudzu. Stir until thickened.

Especially good when used with stir-fried vegetables including red and green bell pepper and carrots. Colorful and tasty!

ALKALINE-STARCH BREADS

Since yeasted bread is hard to digest, the best breads for getting well are the flat breads or sourdough. Whole grains, of course. I have tried many times, with no success, to create a good sourdough rye bread. Mine end up like bricks. Perhaps you can find a whole grain, sourdough bakery.

Tortillas, both corn and whole wheat, are okay, or if you are sensitive to either of those, make your own flat breads with oat or barley flour, a combination of both, or garbanzo flour.

Also, baking soda can cause stomach problems and although baking powder is a little better, but be sure and use the kind without aluminum.

There are also, unyeasted crisp breads available in grocery stores.

Chapati (Flat Bread)

2 cups of whole wheat flour (or 1 cup of oat flour and 1 cup of
    barley flour)
1/2 cup unhulled sesame seeds, finely ground
10 to 12 tablespoons water
1 tablespoon grapeseed oil

1. Mix the flour, sesame and water together. Add oil and knead until smooth.
2. Cut dough in half and divide each half into 6 pieces.
3. Roll each piece into a ball and, on a floured surface, roll pieces into thin 6-inch circles with a rolling pin.
4. Cook on a hot ungreased, cast-iron skillet for about 1 minute, each side.

Makes 12.

Garbanzo Chapati

2 cups garbanzo (chick pea) flour
2/3 cup water
2 teaspoons oil
1 teaspoon sea salt

1. Combine all ingredients and roll into circles as in wheat chapati recipe.
2. Heat a lightly oiled skillet until very hot, then on medium high heat cook each chapati on both sides, about 2 minutes (until slightly brown). Serve warm.

Makes 12.

These can be stored in the refrigerator and lightly toasted later.

Rye Flatbreads

2 cups rye flour
1/2 teaspoon salt
2 teaspoons baking powder
2 tablespoons oil
2/3 cup oat or rice milk

1. Spray and flour 2 baking sheets. Heat oven to 400 degrees.
2. Mix first 3 ingredients together.
3. Mix in oil and milk to make a stiff dough, using your hands to make a ball of dough.
4. Knead on a floured board until smooth. (About 5 minutes.)
5. Divide into 6 pieces and roll each very thin, less than 1/8" thick.
6. Place flatbreads on baking sheets and prick all over with a fork.
7. Bake for 12 to 15 minutes. Cool on a rack.

Makes 6.

Corn Bread

1 3/4 cups cornmeal (roasted)
3 cups boiling water
1/2 cup barley flour
1/3 cup oat flour
1 1/2 cups cooked millet
2 tablespoons grapeseed oil
1 teaspoon Herbamare

To roast cornmeal stir in a skillet over medium heat until it smells like roasted corn.

1. Heat oven to 375 degrees.
2. Transfer cornmeal to a bowl and pour boiling water in, stirring to mix. Let stand, covered for about 10 minutes.
3. Add the rest of the ingredients to the soaked cornmeal, mixing well.
4. Oil a 2-quart baking dish and pour in the batter. Bake for 45 minutes.

Makes 12 pieces.

Sesame Bread Sticks

2 cups of whole wheat flour (or a combination of oat and barley)
1/2 cup sesame seeds
2 teaspoons honey
1/2 teaspoon salt
1/8 cup grapeseed oil
3/4 cup water

1. Heat oven to 350 degrees.
2. Put flour in a bowl and stir in sesame seeds.
3. Combine honey, salt, oil, and water. Stir into flour and mix well. Knead until smooth.
4. Roll into breadstick shapes about 8 inches long by 1/2-inch in diameter.
5. Place on an oiled baking sheet. Bake for about 30 minutes, until golden brown.

Makes 6 to 8.

Mexican Corn Bread

1 cup corn meal
1 cup whole wheat pastry flour
2 teaspoons baking powder
1/2 teaspoon salt
1/2 cup corn kernels
1 small can minced green chiles
1 cup oat milk
1/4 cup oil
1 teaspoon honey

1. Heat oven to 425 degrees. Oil muffin tins.
2. Combine first 4 ingredients in a large bowl.
3. In another bowl, combine the rest of ingredients. Pour wet into dry and stir just until dry mixture is wet.
4. Spoon into muffin tins and bake for 25 to 30 minutes.

Makes 6.

Corn Crisps

2 cups cornmeal
1/2 teaspoon salt
1 1/2 cups boiling water
3 tablespoons of oil

1. Heat oven to 400 degrees. Spray with oil and flour 2 baking sheets.
2. Combine cornmeal and salt in a bowl.
3. Stir in boiling water and let stand for several minutes, until water is absorbed.
4. Stir in oil.
5. Using a tablespoon, drop batter on a sprayed baking sheet, spreading each into thin, 3" rounds.
6. Bake until crisps are golden, about 15 minutes. Serve hot.

Makes about 2 dozen.

Whole Wheat Biscuits

3 cups whole wheat pastry flour
1/2 cup grapeseed oil
4 teaspoons baking powder
1 1/2 teaspoons Herbamare
2/3 cup oat milk

1. Heat oven to 425 degrees.
2. Mix first 4 ingredients together, then stir in the milk.
3. Knead on a lightly floured board for 2 or 3 minutes.
4. Roll or pat out into 1/2" thick dough.
5. Cut rounds with a glass or cutter and place on an oiled baking sheet.
6. Bake for about 15 minutes.

Makes about 9 biscuits.

Oatmeal Crackers

4 cups quick oats
1 cup corn meal
1 cup whole wheat or barley flour
1 3/4 cup unbleached flour
1 cup grapeseed oil
3/4 cup honey
1 1/2 teaspoons salt
Pure water
Sesame seeds

1. Heat oven to 300 degrees
2. Mix oats, cornmeal and flours together
3. Add oil, honey, and salt and add just enough water to make a stiff dough.
4. Knead for 5 minutes, adding sesame seeds to taste.
5. Roll very thin, prick with a fork and mark squares with a knife.
6. Bake on oiled baking sheets for about 25 minutes, or until golden brown.
7. Let cool on a rack, then break into squares and store.

Makes about 4 dozen crackers.

Lemon-Poppy Seed Muffins

Grated peel of two lemons
1/4 cup lemon juice
1/2 cup apple juice
1/2 cup corn oil
1/2 cup maple syrup
1/3 cup poppy seeds
1 cup oat flour
1 cup whole wheat pastry flour
2 teaspoons baking powder
1/2 teaspoon sea salt

1. Heat oven to 375 degrees. Spray muffin tins.
2. Grate and squeeze lemons.
3. Combine lemon peel, lemon juice, apple juice, corn oil, and maple syrup.
4. In a separate bowl, mix together all the rest of the ingredients.
5. Combine wet ingredients with the dry mixture and stir to a smooth batter.
6. Pour batter into muffin cups and bake for 15 minutes. Reduce oven to 350 degrees and bake another 20 minutes.

Makes about 6 muffins.

Apricot-Millet Muffins

1 1/2 cups whole wheat pastry flour
3 teaspoons baking powder
2/3 cup cooked millet
1/2 teaspoon salt
1 cup orange juice
1/2 cup chopped dried apricots
1/3 cup oil
1 tablespoon honey

1. Heat oven to 400 degrees. Oil muffin tins
2. Mix the first 4 ingredients in a large bowl.
3. In another bowl, mix the rest of the ingredients.
4. Combine wet and dry ingredients, mixing just until dry ingredients are wet.
5. Spoon into muffin tins and bake for about 20 minutes. (Until a toothpick, inserted, comes out clean).

Makes about 6 muffins.

DESSERTS

Please use this section sparingly. If you absolutely *must* have sweets, try to eat them apart from meals. At tea time, in the afternoon would be best. I've included several different recipes in the hope that each of you will find one you like. These are so much better for you than the white flour, white sugar, and butter sweets widely available, but they are still not something you should consume frequently.

Baked Apple

4 large cooking apples
1/4 cup maple syrup
1/4 cup raisins
1/2 teaspoon cinnamon
1 cup water

1. Heat oven to 350 degrees.
2. Core apples, leaving 1/4 inch in the base of the apple to hold the filling
3. Place apples in an 8" square baking dish
4. In a small bowl, combine maple syrup, raisins and cinnamon. Mix well.
5. Spoon mixture into the apple cavities
6. Pour the water into the bottom of the baking dish and bake for 1 hour.

Serves 4.

The water will make a syrup that can be spooned over the apples. Serve warm or cold.

Rome Beauty, Johnathan or Fuji are all good baking apples.

Pineapple-Ginger Sorbet

2 15 1/4-ounce cans crushed pineapple in natural juice
1 1/2 tablespoons grated fresh ginger
2 tablespoons maple syrup, or to taste

1. Remove pineapple from cans and spoon into individual ice trays. Freeze until solid
2. About 10 minutes before serving, remove trays from the freezer and let stand at room temperature.
3. In a food processor, combine ginger and maple syrup. Adding a few cubes of pineapple at a time, process until smooth. Serve immediately.

Serves 4.

Oat Pie Crust

1 1/2 cups rolled oats
1/2 cup oat flour (to make oat flour, simply put oats in a blender and blend)
1/4 teaspoon salt
2 tablespoons honey
2 tablespoons apple juice
1/4 cup canola or grapeseed oil

1. Heat oven to 375 degrees and oil a 9" pie pan
2. In a food processor, process rolled oats to a coarse meal.
3. In a bowl, combine processed oats, flour, and salt.
4. In another bowl, combine the rest of the ingredients.
5. Pat into pie pan. Prick with a fork and bake for 15 minutes, or until light golden brown. Fill with any of the following fruit puddings or apple pie filling.

Serves 6 to 8.

Vanilla Pudding

6 cups of oat milk
1 cup of millet
1/3 cup of honey
1/2 teaspoon salt
1/4 cup agar-agar flakes
2 teaspoons vanilla extract

1. Combine ingredients in a sauce pan and bring to a boil. Lower heat and simmer for 30 minutes.
2. Remove from heat and cool.
3. Stir in vanilla and, in batches, purée in a processor until smooth and creamy.
4. Blend batches together and pour into pie shells or pudding cups.

Peach Cream Pie

Prepare the Vanilla Pudding recipe. Bake two 9" pie shells.

4 fresh, ripe peaches, peeled and sliced
2 tablespoons lemon juice
1/8 cup honey

1. Combine lemon juice and honey. Pour over peaches and stir to coat slices.
2. Pour vanilla pudding into the pie shells.
3. Arrange peach slices on top. Chill.

Strawberry or Blueberry Cream Pie

Prepare the Vanilla Pudding recipe.
Bake two 9-inch pie shells.
For Strawberry Cream Pie, simply arrange strawberry halves on top of the pudding.

For Blueberry Topping:
4 cups blueberries
1/2 cup water
1/8 cup honey
2 tablespoons arrowroot dissolved in 1/4 cup cold water

1. In a saucepan, combine blueberries, water, and honey. Bring to a boil and simmer for 5 minutes.
2. Stir in arrowroot mixture and continue simmering until mixture thickens.
3. Cool, then pour on top of the pudding.

Chill both kinds of pie before serving.

"Apple Pie" Filling

4 organic apples (If not organic, peel)
2 cups unsweetened apple juice
1/2 cup raisins
1 cup apple sauce
1 teaspoon cinnamon
1/2 teaspoon coriander
1 tablespoon arrowroot dissolved in
2 tablespoons of water
1 teaspoon vanilla extract

1. Core and slice apples.
2. Put in a saucepan with the apple juice and the raisins. Bring to a boil, lower heat, and simmer for 15 minutes.
3. Stir cinnamon and coriander into the applesauce, then combine it with the cooked apple mixture.
4. Stir in the dissolved arrowroot, and bring the mixture back to a boil, stirring until heated through and thickened
5. Remove from heat and stir in vanilla.
6. Use to fill crepes or spoon into the oat pie crust.

Serves 6 to 8.

Crepes

1 cup oat flour
1 cup barley flour
1/4 teaspoon sea salt
1 1/2 cups unsweetened apple juice (more if needed to result in a
    thin batter).
1 teaspoon vanilla extract

1. Combine flours and salt. Add juice to get a thin,
    pancake-like batter.
2. Stir in vanilla and let sit for an hour or so, if possible.
3. Very lightly oil a skillet (or use a non-stick skillet)
4. When skillet is hot (a drop of water on it will sizzle and
    jump), pour 1/4 cup of batter into the skillet, circling as
    you pour to get it as thin as possible.
5. Cook on medium-high heat until holes begin to appear on
    the surface. Flip the crepe over and cook about half
    a minute.
6. Place each crepe, stacked, in a warm oven until all the
    crepes are cooked.
7. Top each crepe with the cherry sauce or other fruit filling.

Serves 4.

Cherry Sauce

2 cups of frozen pitted cherries (or fresh, in season)
3/4 cup of apple juice
1 tablespoon arrowroot dissolved in
2 tablespoons cold water
1 teaspoon vanilla extract

1. Put cherries and apple juice in a sauce pan. Bring to a boil, lower heat, cover, and simmer for 5 minutes.
2. Stir the arrowroot mixture into the cherries and cook until thickened.
3. Stir in the vanilla extract. Cool.

Use on crepes, on cake, or on vanilla pudding. Or combine crepes, sauce and vanilla pudding for a fancier feast.

Pear Crisp

4 ripe pears, peeled and sliced
1/4 cup raisins
1/8 cup honey
1/2 teaspoon cinnamon
1/2 teaspoon vanilla extract
1 cup rolled oats
3 tablespoons oat flour
1 tablespoon butter, melted
1 tablespoon Sucanat or Fructose

1. Heat oven to 325 degrees and spray an 8" square baking dish.
2. Combine pears, raisins, honey, cinnamon, and vanilla in a bowl. Mix gently.
3. Spoon into the baking dish.
4. Combine oats, flour, butter, and Sucanat and mix well. Spoon on top of pear mixture and bake for 45 minutes. Serve warm or chilled.

Serves 6.

Plain Cake

1 1/4 cup oat flour
1 cup whole wheat pastry flour
2 teaspoons baking powder
1/2 teaspoon salt
1/3 cup grapeseed oil
1/3 cup applesauce
1/4 cup honey
1/4 cup maple syrup
1 1/4 cup water
2 teaspoons vanilla extract

1. Heat oven to 375 degrees and oil a cake pan.
2. Mix dry ingredients together, mixing thoroughly.
3. In a separate bowl, whisk liquid ingredients together.
4. Slowly stir liquid mixture into dry.
5. Pour into cake pan and bake for about 30 minutes (until a toothpick comes out clean).
6. Cool on a rack.

Serves 6.

Prepare any of the following sauces to serve with the cake.

Raspberry Sauce

1 one-pound package frozen or fresh raspberries
2 cups white grape juice or apple juice
2 teaspoons honey
arrowroot

1. Put raspberries and juice in a sauce pan and bring to a boil. Lower heat, cover and simmer for about 8 minutes.
2. Remove from heat and put raspberries in small batches through a wire mesh strainer by pressing with a spoon to remove seeds. (It helps to rinse the strainer occasionally to get rid of the seeds).
3. Measure amount of fruit purée and juice as you return it to the saucepan.
4. Add the honey.
5. For every 1/2 cup of mixture you will need 1 teaspoon of arrowroot dissolved in a small amount of water. Stir the arrowroot mixture into the raspberry mixture.
6. Return to the heat, bringing it back to simmer. Cook, stirring, until thick. Store in refrigerator until ready to use.

Strawberry Sauce

1 pound fresh or frozen strawberries (unsweetened)
2 cups white grape juice or apple juice
2 1/2 tablespoons arrowroot
1/4 cup water
1 teaspoon vanilla extract

1. Put strawberries and juice in a saucepan. Bring to a boil, reduce heat, cover and simmer for about 10 minutes.
2. Dissolve arrowroot in water and stir into the strawberries. Cook, stirring, until thickened.
3. Stir in vanilla. Cool. Refrigerate.

Fresh Blueberry Sauce

1 pint fresh blueberries
1 1/2 teaspoons lemon zest
1/8 cup maple syrup

In a food processor, combine all ingredients and process until creamy. Use on top of cake or pour sauce on dessert plates and top with fruit of your choice. Can also be used on crepes.

Resources

Alternative Medical Associations:

Naturopathy:
American Association of Naturopathic Physicians
601 Valley Street, Suite 105 Seattle, WA 98109
    1-206-298-0125
http: //www.infinite.org/naturopathic.physician

American Naturopathic Medical Assoc.
P.O. Box 96273
Las Vegas, NV 89193
    1-702-897-7053
http: //www.anma.corn

Homeopathic:
National Center for Homeopathy
801 N. Fairfax St., Suite 306
Alexandria, VA 22314
    1-703-548-7790
http: //www.homeopathic.org

International Foundation for Homeopathy
P.O. Box 7
Edmonds, WA 98020
    1-425-776-4147
http: //www.net/ifh

Hypnosis:

American Board of Hypnotherapy
16842 Von Karman Ave, Suite 475
Irvine, CA 92606
1-800-872-9996
http: //www.hypnosis.com

The American Society of Clinical Hypnosis
2200 East Devon Ave., Suite 291
Des Plaines, IL 60018
1-847-297-3317
http: //www.asch.net

National Guild of Hypnotists
P.O. Box 308
Merrimack, NH 03054
1-603-429-9438
http: //www.nghhq@aol .com

Massage/Bodywork:

American Massage Therapy Assoc.
820 Davis Street, Suite 100
Evanston, IL 60201-4444
1-847-864-0123

Associated Bodywork & Massage Professionals
28677 Buffalo Park Road
Evergreen, CO 80439-7347
1-800-458-2267
http: //www.abmp.com

International Massage Association
3000 Connecticut Ave. N.W., Suite 308
Washington, DC 20008
1-202-387-6555
http: //www.imagroup.com

Holistic Medicine:

American Holistic Medical Assoc.
6728 Old McLean Village Drive
McLean, VA 22101
http: //www.ahmaholistic.com

The Mind/Body Medical Institute
Beth Israel Deaconess Medical Center,
Division of Behavioral Medicine
100 Francis Street, Suite 1A
Boston, MA 02215
    1-617-632-9525
http: //www.med.harvard.edu/programs/mind/body

Aromatherapy:

National Association for Holistic Aromatherapy
219 Carl Street
San Francisco, CA 94117-3804
    1-415-564-6785

Ayurvedic/Indian Medicine:

American Institute of Ayurvedic Sciences
2115 112th Ave. N.E.
Bellevue, WA 98004
    1-425-453-8022
http: //www.ayurvedicscience.com

The Ayurvedic Institute
P.O. Box 23445
Albuquerque, NM 87192-1445
    1-505-291-9698

American Academy of Environmental Medicine
4510 W. 89th St. #110
Prairie Village, KS 66207
   1-913-248-0067
(Send a SASE for a list of alternative doctors in your area)

American Academy of Environmental Medicine
10 Randolph St.
New Hope, PA 18938
   1-215-862-4544
http: //www.aaem.com

Acupuncture:

American Academy of Medical Acupuncture
5820 Wilshire Blvd., Suite 500
Los Angeles, CA 90036
   1-800-521-2262
(To locate a physician qualified to practice acupuncture near you.)

Acupressure:

American Oriental Bodywork Therapy Assoc.
Laurel Oak Corporate Center, Suite 408
1010 Haddonfield-Berlin Rd.
Voorhees, NJ 08043
   1-609-782-1616

Oriental Medicine:

American Association of Oriental Medicine
433 Front Street
Catasauqua, PA 18032
   1-610-266-1433

Biofeedback:

Biofeedback Certification Institute of America
10200 West 44th Ave., Suite 304
Wheat Ridge, CO 80033-2840
1-303-420-2902

Chiropractic:

American Chiropractic Association
1701 Clarendon Blvd.
Arlington, VA 22209
1-703-276-8800
http: //www.amerchiro.org

International Chiropractors Association
1110 North Blebe Road, Suite 1000
Arlington, VA 22201
1-800-423-4690
http: //www.chiropractic.org

Energy Medicine:

International Society for the Study of Subtle Energies
and Energy Medicine
356 Goldco Circle
Golden, CO 80403
1-303-425-4625
http: //www.vitalenergy.com/issseem/.

Osteopathy:

American Osteopathic Association
142 East Ontario Street
Chicago, IL 60611
1-800-621-1773
http: //www.amosteo-assn.org.

Polarity Therapy:

American Polarity Therapy Assoc.
2888 Bluff Street, Suite 149
Boulder, CO 80301
    1-800-359-5620
http: //www.polaritytherapy.org

Reflexology:

International Institute of Reflexology
P.O. Box 12642
St. Petersburg, FL 33733-2642
    1-813-343-4811

Reiki:

The Reiki Alliance
P.O. Box 41
Cataldo, ID 83810
    1-208-682-3535

Therapeutic Touch:

Nurse Healers-Professional Associates
1211 Locust Street
Philadelphia, PA 19107
    1-215-545-8079
http: //www.therapeutic-touch.org

Flower Essences:

Flower Essence Society
P.O. Box 1769
Nevada City, CA 95959
    1-916-265-0258
http: //www.floweressence.com

Music Therapy:

American Music Therapy Association
8455 Colesville Road, Suite 1000
Silver Spring, NY 20910
   1-301-589-3300
http: //www.rnusictherapy.org

Multiple Sclerosis Researcher Hans Nieper, M.D. has a program to follow. For details on the Nieper program contact:

AK Brewer Science Library
325 N. Central Avenue
Richland Center, WI 53581
   Fax #: 608-647-6797

For the Calcium EAP supplement recommended by Dr. Nieper:

BioResource Inc
Box 2352
Santa Rosa, CA 95405
   1-800-203-3775

Special Information on MS:

Swank Clinic
13655 S.W. Jenkins Road
Beaverton, OR 97005
   1-503-520-1015
   Fax: 1-503-520-1223
E-mail: swank@involved.com

Health-related web sites:

Acupuncture:
http: //www.acupuncture.com

Alternative Medicine Digest:
http: //www.alternativemedicine.com

Aromatherapy:
http: //www.geocities.com/-aromaweb/index.html

Bodywise:
http: //www.bodywise.net

HealthWorld Online:
http: //www.healthy.net

HealthWWWeb:
http: //www.healthwwweb.com

Healthy Ideas:
http: //www.prevention.com

HerbNet:
http: //www.herbnet.com

Homeopathy Home Page:
http: //www.cambr. force9 .co.uk

Nutrition:
http: //www.cyberdiet.com

Oriental Medicine:
http: //www.aaom.org

Public Medicine:
http: //www.ncbi.nlm.nih.gov/PubMed

Sapient Health Network:
http: //www.shn.net/corp.html

Vegetarian Resource Group:
http://www.vrg.org

Wellness Web:
http: //www.wellweb.com

Alternative Health Newsletters:

Dr. David Williams
Alternatives
P.O. Box 829
Ingram, TX 78025
1-800-5273044

Dr. Christiane Northrup's
Health Wisdom for Women
7811 Montrose Road
Potomac, MD 20854
1-800-804-0935

Health Sciences Institute
105 W. Monument Street
P.O. Box 17560
Baltimore, MD 21298
1-800-981-7157

Dr. Julian Whitaker's Health & Healing
Phillips Publishing Inc.
P.O. Box 60042
7811 Montrose Road
Potomac, MD 20859-0042
1-800-539-8219

Dr. Robert Atkins' Health Revelations
Agora Health Publishing
105 West Momument St.
Baltimore, MD 21201
1-410-895-7900

Dr. Andrew Weil's Self Healing
42 Pleasant St.
Watertown, MA 02172
1-800-523-3296

Supplements:

The Vitamin Shoppe
1-800-223-1216
Call for a catalogue
www.vitaminshoppe.com

Probiotics:

Nutrition Now
1-800-929-0418
http://www. nutritionnow.com
LIFESTAR International. Inc
Advanced Nutritional Systems
San Francisco, CA 94103

Foods:

Adobe Mill Company
P.O. Box 596
Dove Creek, CO 81324
1-800-ADOBE
Dried beans, blue cornmeal, spices

Allergy Resource
195 Huntington Beach Drive
Colorado Springs, CO 80921
1-719-488-3630
Wheat free and gluten free products

American Spood Foods
P.O. Box 566
Petoskey, MI 49770
 1-800-222-5886
Dried cherries, other fruits, sugarless preserves

Arrowhead Mills, Inc.
P.O. Box 2059
Hereford, TX 79045
 1-806-364-0730
Whole grains, flours, beans, tahini, oils, etc.

Aux Delices des Bois
4 Leonard Street
New York, NY 10013
 1-212-334-1230
Fresh and dried mushrooms

Berkshire Mountain Bakery
P.O. Box 785
Housatonic, MA 01236
 1-800-274-3412

Big Flavor Foods, Inc.
P.O. Box 331597
Miami, FL 33233
 1-800-352-8670
Santa Fe Smoke, Hanoi Hot and other spice mixes

Chukar Cherry Company
320 Wine Country Rd.
P.O. Box 510
Prosser, WA 99350
 1-800-624-9544
Dried fruit

Dean & Deluca, Inc
560 Broadway
New York, NY 10012
   1-800-221-7714
Oils, vinegars, beans, Puys lentils and other exotic beans

DeWildt Imports, Inc.
RD 3, Fox Gap Road
Bangor, PA 18013
   1-800-338-3433
Asian ingredients and cookware

Diamond Organics
Freedom, CA 95019
   1-800-922-2396
Organic greens and vegetables

Eden Foods
701 Tecumseh
Clifton, MI 49236
   1-517-456-7424
Organic pastas, sea vegetables, grains, vinegars, shoyu, etc.

Earl Ebersol Farms
27828 S.W. 127th Ave.
Homestead, FL 33032
Citrus fruits

En-R-G Foods, Inc.
P.O. Box 84487
Seattle, WA 98124
   1-800-331-5222
Wheat free-gluten free

Fantastic Foods
106 Galli Drive
Novato, CA 94949
   1-415-883-7718
Healthful instant foods!

Flora Source
1-800-780-1198 ext. 283
Golden Health Products Inc.
6 Kentucky Road
Quincy, IL 62301

Fox Hill Farm
444 West Michigan Ave.
P.O. Box 79
Parma, MI 49269
1-517-531-3179
Ships fresh herbs

French Meadow Bakery
2601 Lyndale Ave. South
Minneapolis, MN 55972
1-612-870-4740

Granary Natural Foods Market
1400 Main Street
Suite 207
Sarasota, FL 34236
1-800-274-2749
Over 15,000 items. Catalog.

Gold Mine Natural Food Co.
1947 30th Street
San Diego, CA 92102
1-800-457-FOOD
Macrobiotic Specialties (No minimum order)

Lunberg Family Farms
P.O. Box 369
Richvale, CA 95974
1-916-882-4551
Organic rice, rice syrup, rice cakes and RizCous

Morinaga Nutritional Foods, Inc.
5800 Eastern Avenue
Suite 270
Los Angeles, CA 90040
    1-213-728-4325
Aseptically packaged silken tofu

Mountain Ark Trading Company
P.O. Box 1037
Fayetteville, AR 72702
    1-800-643-8909
Everything from grains to cookware. (Mac knives). A great variety!

Nasoya Foods Ind.
23 Jytek Drive
Leominster, MA 01453
    1-508-537-0713
Tofu and Nayonaise, a tofu based mayonnaise

Nature's Herb Company
1010 46th Street
Emeryville, CA 94608
    1-800-227-2830
Agar by the pound at reasonable prices

Northern Soy, Inc.
545 West Avenue
Rochester, NY 14611
    1-716-235-8970
A really good soy "hot dog," Not Dog and vegetarian breakfast
link sausages

Oasis Breads
440 Venture Street
P.O. Box 182
Escondido, CA 92025
    1-619-747-7390
Sourdough bread, etc.

Ocean Harvest
P.O. Box 1719
Mendocino, CA 95460
   1-707-964-7869
Sea vegetables, including a very special one called sea palm.

Once Again Nut Butters, Inc.
12 State Street
Nunda, NY 14517
   1-716-468-2535
Lots of nut butters and tahini

Sovex Natural Foods, Inc.
P.O. Box 310
Collegedale, TN 37315
   1-615-396-3145
Hickory smoked yeast with a bacon-like flavor.

Soyco Foods
Northgate Industrial Park
R.D. #3
P.O. Box 5204
New Castle, PA 16105
   1-412-656-1102
Soy cheese called Soymage

Spectrum Naturals
133 Copeland Street
Petaluma, CA 94952
   1-707-778-8900
Wide selection of oils and educational materials about oils.

Spice of Life
P.O. Box 1287
Fallbrook, CA 92028
   1-619-237-3677
Herbs and herb blends that are not irradiated.

Taylor's Herb Gardens
1535 Lone Oak Road
Vista, CA 92083
　1-714-727-3485
Fresh herbs and herbs and seeds to grow yourself.

Vogue Cuisine, Inc.
437 Golden Isles Drive
Suite 15 G
Hallandale, FL 33009
　1-305-458-2915
Vogue Vege Base, a great seasoning for vegetarians

Walnut Acres Organic Farms
Walnut Acres Rd.
Penns Creek, PN 17862
　1-800-433-3998

Williams-Sonoma
100 North Point Street
San Francisco, CA 94133
　1-415-421-4242

Suggested reading:

Mysterious Causes & Cures of Illness
Dr. Jonn Matsen, N.D.
Fischer Publishing

Food and Healing
Annemarie Colbin
Ballantine Books

Prescription for Nutrional Healing
James Balch, M.D. & Phyllis Balch
Avery Publishing Group
(Has a great reference section!)

The Macrobiotic Way
Michio Kushi
Avery Publishing Group

Behavioral Kinesiology
John Diamond, M.D.
Harper & Row, Publishers

Body Reflexology
Mildred Carter
Parker Publishing Company

Your Body Doesn't Lie
John Diamond, M.D.
Warner Books

5-Day Allergy Relief System
Dr. Marshall Mandell &
Lynne Scanion
Pocket Books

Super Immunity
Paul Pearsall, Ph.D.
Fawcett Gold Medal

The Healing Power of Mind
Tulku Thondup
Shambhala

Enter The Zone & Mastering The Zone
Barry Sears Ph.D.
Regan Books

Magazines:

Natural Health. For subscription inquiries: 1-800-526-8440

Vegetarian Times. For subscription inquiries: 1-800-829-3340

Index

Acid foods, 94, 115.
    See also Acid-Protein foods
Acid-Protein foods
  appetizers, 124-128
  desserts, 196-198
  egg dishes, 162-167
  examples of, 115
  recipe listing, 117-120
  salads, 137-147
  sauces and gravies, 191-195
  seafood, 168-181
  soups, 129-136
  vegetables, 182-190
Acorn Squash Purée, 245
acupressure, 274
acupuncture, 10-11, 61, 274, 277
Aduki Bean Dip, 220
aduki beans, 107
agar-agar, 81, 107
Airola, Paavo, 5-6
Alkaline-Starch foods
  appetizers, 219-224
  breads, 253-260
  combining, 94
  desserts, 123, 261-270
  salads, 122, 232-240
  sandwiches, 241
  sauces, 250-252
  soups, 225-231
  vegetables, 242-249
alkalizing foods, 70

allergies, 11
almond recipes
  almond cream, 135
  Almond Ginger Sauce, 191
  almond milk, 107
  Almond Pesto, 171
  almonds, blanched, 187
  Broiled Fish with Almond Pesto, 171
  Butterscotch Mousse with
     Toasted Almonds, 196
  Curried Tofu, 157
  Deviled Crab, 175
  Green Beans Almondine, 187
aloe vera, 48
alternative medicine
    associations, 271, 278
alternative medicine
    newsletters, 279-280
American Medical Association
    (AMA), 61-63
appetizer recipes
  Aduki Bean Dip, 220
  Baked Garlic on Toast, 224
  Carrot Paté, 221
  Garlic-Ripe Olive Dip, 124
  Guacamole-Tofu Dip, 128
  Lentil Paté, 219
  Little Protein Dippers, 126
  Mushroom Crostini, 223
  Quick Guacamole, 128
  Red Bell Pepper Dip, 222

Roasted Garbanzo Beans, 223
Roasted Red Pepper Dip, 199
Roasted Sweet Onion and
    Garlic Spread, 224
Tofu-Onion Dip, 127
Vegetable Plate, 199
Warm Artichoke Dip, 125
White Bean Paté, 222
apple recipes
  Apple Pie Filling, 265
  Baked Apple, 261
  Stuffed Squash, 248
applied kinesiology, 113-114
Apricot-Millet Muffins, 260
arachidonic acid, 53, 108
aromatherapy, 105, 273, 278
arrowroot, 81, 107
arthritis, 48, 70
artichoke recipes
  Fish with Artichokes, 170
  Tuna Casserole, 178
  Warm Artichoke Dip, 125
artificial sweeteners, 75
asparagus recipes
  Asparagus Quiche Sans Crust, 149
  Cream of Asparagus Soup, 134
aspartame, 75
astragalus, 49-50
Atkins, Dr. Robert, 279
attitude, importance of, 40
autoimmune diseases, 51-52
avocado recipes
  Carrot Paté, 221
  Cool Avocado Soup, 202
  Guacamole-Tofu Dip, 128
  Quick Guacamole, 128
  Spinach Salad with Dijon
      Dressing, 140
Ayurvedic/Indian medicine, 273

Baked Apple, 261
Baked Carrots and Onions, 214
Baked Garlic on Toast, 224
Baked Garlic Potatoes, 246
Baked Potato Soup, 225

Baked Whitefish with Horseradish-
    Mayonnaise, 170
Balsamic Glazed Onions, 210
balsamic vinegar, 107-108
Barbecue Sauce, 195
Barbequed Salmon, 176
barley grass juice, 49
Beets, Dilled Baby, 209
Beet Sauce, Beautiful, 251
bee venom, 66
bell pepper recipes.
    See also red bell pepper recipes
Benge, Charles, 89-91
biofeedback, 275
biotherapy, 46
Black Bean Soup, 230
Blackened Tofu, 152
black-eyed pea recipes
  Black-Eyed Pea-Sweet Potato
      Salad, 234
  Texas Caviar, 236
blood clotting, 47
blood sugar, 56
blood tests, 33
Blueberry Cream Pie, 264
Blueberry Sauce, 270
bodywork (massage), 11, 39, 272
borage oil, 53
bovine growth hormone, 77
brain tumor diagnosis, 9-10
Braised Red Cabbage, 243
bread recipes. See also muffin recipes
  Chapati, 253
  Corn Bread, 255
  Corn Crisps, 257
  Garbanzo Chapati, 254
  Mexican Corn Bread, 256
  Rye Flatbreads, 254
  Sesame Bread Sticks, 256
  Whole Wheat Biscuits, 257
broccoli recipes
  Broccoli Casserole, 189
  Broccoli-Red Pepper Stir-Fry, 186
  Broccoli-Soy Cheese Soup, 129
  Broccoli-Tofu Souffle, 151
  Chinese Quinoa Salad, 240

Index

Creamy Veggie Bake, 156
Garlic Green Broccoli, 214
Oriental Broccoli Quiche
   Sans Crust, 148
   steaming, 199
Broiled Fish with Almond Pesto, 171
Brown Mushroom Sauce, 250
Brussels Sprouts, Savory, 182
burdock root, 24
butter, 80
Butternut Squash-Orange Purée, 242
Butterscotch Mousse with
   Toasted Almonds, 196

cabbage recipes
   Braised Red Cabbage, 243
   Healing Vegetable Soup, 228
   Oriental Salad, 146, 205
   Quick Steamed Vegetable Soup, 202
   Southwest Slaw, 207
   Steamed Cabbage, 215
Caesar Crab Salad, 137
Caesar Salad, 138
caffeine, 75-76
Cake, Plain, 268
calcium citrate, 52
calcium EAP, 52, 277
cancer and diet, 52
candida (yeast), 28, 35-36
Canned-Tuna Bake, 181
canola oil, 80
capsicum (cayenne), 48, 49
carbohydrate intake, 56-58
carob, 80
Carrot Paté, 221
carrot recipes
   Baked Carrots and Onions, 214
   Carrot Paté, 221
   Carrots, Zucchini and Peas, 215
   Carrots with Coriander, 212
   Four Color Stir-Fry, 209
   Golden Bisque, 230
   Pineapple-Glazed Carrots, 242
   Puréed Carrot Soup, 203
cashew recipes
   Broccoli-Soy Cheese Soup, 129

Butterscotch Mousse with
   Toasted Almonds, 196
   cashew cream, 156
   Cashew-Ginger Sauce, 194
   Cashew Sauce, 191
   Garlic-Ripe Olive Dip, 124
   Mocha Mousse with
      Toasted Pecans, 198
   Shrimp-Cashew Szechuan Stir Fry, 177
   Tofu-Onion Dip, 127
   Warm Artichoke Dip, 125
   Zucchini with Ginger and Cashews, 183
cat's claw, 49
cauliflower recipes
   Cauliflower with Peanut Sauce, 188
   Four Color Stir-Fry, 209
   Tofu-Cauliflower Casserole, 160
cayenne, 48, 49
Celery Soup, Quick Cream of, 231
Chapati, 253-254
chemotherapy, 19-20, 25
Cherry Sauce, 267
chewing food, importance of, 86-87
Chinese Quinoa Salad, 240
chin lowering, 6
chiropractic, 11, 61, 275
chlorophyll, 49-50, 104
chocolate, 76, 80
circulatory system, 48
Citricidal, 50
coconut, 80
coffee, 75
coffee substitutes, 79
cola drinks, 75, 80
Colbin, Annemarie, 43
colds, 50
Complete Meal Quinoa Salad, 232
computer radiation, 104-105
concentration difficulty, 28
Cool Avocado Soup, 202
cornmeal recipes
   Corn Bread, 255
   Corn Crisps, 257
   Mexican Corn Bread, 256
   Oatmeal Crackers, 258

crab recipes
Caesar Crab Salad, 137
Crab and Mushroom Bake, 174
Deviled Crab, 175
Crackers, Oatmeal, 258
cream soups
Cream of Asparagus Soup, 134
Cream of Celery Soup, 231
Cream of Mushroom Soup, 136
Cream of Tomato Soup, 130
Creamy Veggie Bake, 156
Crepes, 266
Crunchy Mexican Salad, 206
Curried Tofu, 157
cytotoxic tests, 33
cytotoxin, 19-20, 25

dairy products, 52, 76-77
deodorants, 110
desserts. *See also* pies and pie crusts
Baked Apple, 261
Butterscotch Mousse, 196
Crepes, 266
Lemon Mousse, 197
Mocha Mousse with
Toasted Pecans, 198
Pear Crisp, 267
Pineapple-Ginger Sorbet, 262
Plain Cake, 268
Vanilla Pudding, 263
The Detox Diet (Haas), 106
detoxification, 62, 105-106
Deviled Crab, 175
Deviled Eggs, 166
diabetes, 76
diet
combining foods, 93-95, 98
cooking for others, 72-73
fruits and vegetables in, 52, 84
individuality of, 55-56, 58
overview, 97-99, 101-106
raw food, 13-14, 16, 20, 57, 116
rotary diversified, 33
digestive enzymes, 49, 88
digestive systems, 85-88
Dijon dressing, 140

Dilled Baby Beets, 209
dips. *See* appetizer recipes
dizziness, 47
doctors, finding the right one, 59-60, 105
dressings
Dijon, 140
ginger, 139
for Great American Green Salad, 204
Green Goddess, 147
Mexican, 206
for Quinoa Salad, 240
ranch, 141
for Southwest Lentil Salad, 235
for Southwest Slaw, 207
for Spanish Rice Salad, 238
for Taco Salad, 237

E. coli bacteria, 48
earthworm compost, 13-14
Eastman, "Doc," 3
echinacea, 49-50
eggs, 108
Eggplant, Pureéd, 185
egg recipes
Basic Omelet, 162
Deviled Eggs, 166
Omelet Variations, 163
Scrambled Eggs, 166
Spanish Omelet Sauce, 164
Vegetable Omelet, 165
Zucchini Pancake, 167
Egg Replacer Silken Omelet, 162
eicosapentaenoic acid (EPA), 53
elderberry, 50
energy in food, 51
energy medicine, 275
environmental medicine, 274
EPA (eicosapentaenoic acid), 53
essential fatty acids, 57
exercise, 103

falling down, 5-6, 8
fasting, 29
fats and oils, 30, 32, 57, 80, 115
fatty foods, 20, 57, 80
Fiber Greens, 49, 52

fish recipes
  Barbecued Salmon, 176
  Broiled Fish with Almond Pesto, 171
  Canned-Tuna Bake, 181
  Fish Chowder, 135
  Fish Dijon, 168
  Fish Fromage, 169
  Fish with Artichokes, 170
  Grilled Tuna with Teriyaki Sauce, 172
  Poached Fish with Mushrooms, 180
  Salmon Patties with
      Mustard Sauce, 179
  Salmon Salad, 143
  Tuna Casserole, 178
  Tuna Salad in Stuffed Tomato, 143
Flat Bread, 253-254
flax oil, 52-53
Flower Essences, 276
flu, 50
food allergies
  commercial food sources, 280-286
  common troublemakers, 113
  discovering, 6, 29, 102, 113-114
  immediate symptoms of, 30
Food and Drug Administration
    (FDA), 44-45
food cravings, 32-33
food diaries, 25, 29-33, 101-102
food preparation, Zen of, 111-112
food products, commercial
    sources, 280-286
foot reflexology, 65-66, 276
Four Color Stir-Fry, 209
Fresh Blueberry Sauce, 270
fruit recipes.
    See under individual fruits
fruits
  Acid, 115
  Alkaline, 116
  ingestion, 51-52, 84, 94

gallbladders, 86
gamma linolenic acid (GLA), 53
garbanzo recipes
  Garbanzo Beans, Roasted, 223
  Garbanzo Chapati, 254

Garbanzo Salad, 234
garlic, 48, 50
garlic recipes
  Baked Garlic on Toast, 224
  Baked Garlic Potatoes, 246
  Garlic Green Beans or Broccoli, 214
  Garlic-Ripe Olive Dip, 124
  Garlic Spread, 224
  Puréed Vegetables with
    Roasted Garlic, 211
gazpacho, 130, 200
ginger, 47-48, 50
ginger recipes
  Almond Ginger Sauce, 191
  Cashew-Ginger Sauce, 194
  Green Salad and Pecans
    with Ginger Dressing, 139
  Orange-Ginger Sauce, 252
  Pineapple-Ginger Sorbet, 262
  Sweet and Sour Sauce, 194
GLA (gamma linolenic acid), 53
Golden Bisque, 230
goldenseal, 49-50
Gordon, Monteen, 47
grains, 56-57, 116
grapeseed oil, 80, 108
gravies, 195, 218. *See also* sauce recipes
gravitational fields, 104
Great American Green Salad, 204
Green Beans, Garlic, 214
Green Beans Almondine, 187
Green Goddess Dressing, 147
Green Magma, 49, 52
Green Salad and Pecans with
    Ginger Dressing, 139
Grilled Tofu Steaks, 158
Grilled Tuna with Teriyaki Sauce, 172
Grilled Vegetable Salad, 142
Guacamole-Tofu Dip, 128
Guide to Alternative Medicine
    (Rosenfeld), 62-63, 114

Haas, Elson, 62, 106
Hahnemann, Samuel, 60
headaches, 47

The Healing Power of Mind
   (Thondup), 40
Healing Vegetable Soup, 228
heartburn, 49
heart disease, 52
Herbamare, 108
hijiki, 24
Hippocrates, 45, 60, 71
Hodgkin's disease, 62
holistic medicine, 273
homeopathy, 35-37, 60, 271, 278
homogenization, 76
horseradish, 88
Horseradish-Mayonnaise, 170
Horseradish-White Bean Salad, 239
hot baths, 10
The How To Herb Book
   (Keith and Gordon), 47
hypnosis, self, 40-41, 102, 272
hypoglycemia, 49. *See also* blood sugar

iatrogenic disease, 67
IgE/RAST tests, 33
immune system
  as the enemy, 19
  strengthening, 35-36
  suppression of, 45-46
"incurable" diagnosis, 17, 37, 40
Indian medicine, 273
indigestion, 49
Indonesian Tofu, 153
insomnia, 66
irritability, 28

jalapeños
  Jalapeño-Dill Sauce, 192
  Southwest Slaw, 207
  Spanish Omelet Sauce, 164
  Texas Caviar, 236

Kale, Stir-Fried with Garlic, 210
kale soup, 228
Keith, Velma J., 47
kelp, 108
knives, 111, 284
kombu, 108

kudzu, 81, 108
Kushi, Aveline, 27
KyoGreen, 52
Kyolic Formula 102, 48

Lactobacillus acidophilus, 104
lactose, 76
laughter, 39
Lemon Mousse, 197
Lemon-Poppy Seed Muffins, 259
Lemon Sauce, 193
Lemon-Tofu Nuggets, 154
lentil recipes
  Lentil Paté, 219
  Lentil Salad, Southwest, 235
  Lentil Soup, 227
Lima Bean Soup, 226
Liquid Aminos, 108
Little Protein Dippers, 126
liver, 85-86
Lou Gehrig's disease, 16-17
lymph system, 86

Macrobiotic Kushi Institute, 27-28
macrobiotics, 23-24, 27-28, 110
Manhattan Fish Chowder, 135
margarine, 80
massage therapy, 11, 39, 272
meal suggestions, 94-95
memory loss, 28
Mexican Corn Bread, 256
milk, 76-77
milk substitutes, 80
Millet-Apricot Muffins, 260
miso, 24, 28
mousse recipes
  Butterscotch Mousse with
    Toasted Almonds, 196
  Lemon Mousse, 197
  Mocha Mousse with
    Toasted Pecans, 198
moxibustion, 24
MRI, 16
MS. *See* multiple sclerosis
muffin recipes
  Apricot-Millet, 260

Index

Lemon-Poppy Seed, 259
multiple sclerosis (MS)
  conventional treatment, 19
  diagnosis, 11, 15-16
  gradual improvement, 36
  gradual onset, 5-6, 8
  information on, 277
  muscle testing
    (applied kinesiology), 113-114
mushroom recipes
  Basic Omelet For Two, 163
  Broccoli Casserole, 189
  Brown Mushroom Sauce, 250
  Crab and Mushroom Bake, 174
  Cream of Mushroom Soup, 136
  Fish with Artichokes, 170
  Mushroom Crostini, 223
  Mushroom Sauce, 216
  Mushroom-Tomato Salad, 145
  Mushroom-Zucchini Puff, 184
  Poached Fish with Mushrooms, 180
  Shrimp Creole, 173
  Tofu Loaf, 158-159
  Tofu-Mushroom Pancake, 155
  Vegetable Omelet, 165
music therapy, 277
Mustard Sauce, 179
myrrh, 49

Nambudripad Allergy Elimination
  Technique (NAET), 33
naturopathy, 60-62, 271
nausea and vomiting, 47
Neutral foods
  appetizers, 199
  combining, 94
  listing, 115-116
  salads, 204-207
  sauces, 216-218
  soups, 200-203
  vegetables, 208-215
Neutral Gazpacho, 200
niacin flushes, 30
Nieper, Hans, M.D., 52, 277
nightshades, 69-70
night sweats, 6

Northrup, Dr. Christiane, 279
No-See-Ums, 21, 50
nut milks, 80-81, 107

oatmeal, 53, 56
Oatmeal Crackers, 258
Oat Pie Crust, 262
obesity, 83
oils and fats, 30, 32, 57, 80, 115
olive oil, 80
omelet recipes, 163-165
Onions, Baked Carrots and, 214
Onions, Balsamic Glazed, 210
Onions, Roasted Sweet, 224
Orange-Ginger Sauce, 252
organic foods, 31, 87-88, 98
Oriental Broccoli Quiche Sans Crust, 148
Oriental medicine, 274, 278
Oriental Salad, 146, 205
osteopathy, 61, 275
osteoporosis, 75

Pancake, Tofu-Mushroom, 155
papaya, 49
Paracelsus, 60
pasteurization, 77
Peach Cream Pie, 263
Peanut Sauce, 188, 192
Pear Crisp, 267
Pecan Gravy, Roasted, 195
People Against Cancer, 90-91
Pesto, Almond, 171
phosphatidyl ethanolamine, 52
phytochemicals, 51
pies and pie crusts
  Apple Pie Filling, 265
  Oat Pie Crust, 262
  Peach Cream Pie, 263
  Strawberry or Blueberry
    Cream Pie, 264
pineapple recipes
  Pineapple-Ginger Sorbet, 262
  Pineapple-Glazed Carrots, 242
  Sweet and Sour Sauce, 252
Plain Cake, 268
Poached Fish with Mushrooms, 180

polarity therapy, 276
Poppy Seed-Lemon Muffins, 259
potato recipes.
    See also sweet potato recipes
Baked Garlic Potatoes, 246
Baked Potato Soup, 225
Scalloped Potatoes, 247
Spiced Mixed Fries, 249
prescription drugs, 44, 45
primrose oil, 53
probiotics, 52, 104, 280
prostate cancer, 89-91
Prostate Specific Antigen (PSA), 89-90
protein, 56, 76.
    See also Acid-Protein foods
Pudding, Vanilla, 263
pulse rate, 30
Puréed Carrot Soup, 203
Pureéd Eggplant, 185
Puréed Vegetables with
    Roasted Garlic, 211

qi energy, 61
quiches
    Asparagus Quiche Sans Crust, 149
    Oriental Broccoli Quiche
        Sans Crust, 148
    Spinach Quiche Sans Crust, 150
Quick Black Bean Soup, 230
Quick Brown Sauce, 217
Quick Cream of Celery Soup, 231
Quick Guacamole, 128
Quick Steamed Vegetable Soup, 202
quinoa recipes
    Chinese Quinoa Salad, 240
    Complete Meal Quinoa Salad, 232
    Quinoa Stir-Fried Vegetable Salad, 233

ranch dressing, 141
Raspberry Sauce, 269
red bell pepper recipes
    Broccoli-Red Bell Pepper Stir Fry, 186
    Four Color Stir-Fry, 209
    Red Bell Pepper Dip, 222
    Red Bell Pepper Sauce, 216
    Roasted Red Pepper Dip, 199

Roasted Vegetables, 213
Red Cabbage, Braised, 243
reflexology, 65-66, 276
Reiki, 276
rheumatoid arthritis, 76
Rice, Spanish, 238
Rigg, Arthur, 7
Roasted Garbanzo Beans, 223
Roasted Garlic, 211, 224
Roasted Pecan Gravy, 195
Roasted Red Pepper Dip, 199
Roasted Sweet Onion and
    Garlic Spread, 224
Roasted Vegetables, 213
rotary diversified diet, 33
Rye Flatbreads, 254

salad recipes
    Black-Eyed Pea-Sweet Potato, 234
    Caesar, 138
    Caesar Crab, 137
    Chinese Quinoa, 240
    Complete Meal Quinoa, 232
    Crunchy Mexican, 206
    Garbanzo, 234
    Great American Green, 204
    Green Goddess Dressing, 147
    Green Salad & Pecans with
        Ginger Dressing, 139
    Grilled Vegetable, 142
    Mushroom-Tomato, 145
    Oriental, 146, 205
    Quinoa Stir-Fried Vegetable, 233
    Salmon, 143
    Shrimp Louis, 144
    Southwest Lentil, 235
    Southwest Slaw, 207
    Spanish Rice, 238
    Spinach Salad with Dijon Dressing, 140
    Taco, 237
    Texas Caviar, 236
    Tuna Salad in Stuffed Tomato, 143
    Vegetable Salad with
        Creamy Ranch Dressing, 141
    White Bean-Horseradish, 239
salmon, 53. *See also* fish recipes

salmon recipes
  Salmon, Barbequed, 176
  Salmon Patties with
    Mustard Sauce, 179
  Salmon Salad, 143
salt, 109
Sambucol, 50
sandwich recipes, 241
saturated fats, 30, 32, 80
sauce recipes
  Almond Ginger, 191
  Barbecue, 195
  Beautiful Beet, 251
  Blueberry, 270
  Brown Mushroom, 250
  Cashew, 191
  Cashew-Ginger, 194
  Cauliflower with Peanut, 188
  Cherry, 267
  Fresh Blueberry, 270
  Grilled Tuna with Teriyaki, 172
  Jalapeño-Dill, 192
  Lemon, 193
  Mushroom, 216
  Mustard, 179
  Orange-Ginger, 252
  Peanut, 188, 192
  Quick Brown, 217
  Raspberry, 269
  Red Bell Pepper, 216
  Salmon Patties with Mustard, 179
  Soy Cheese, 193
  Spanish Omelet, 164
  Stir-Fry, 251
  Strawberry, 269
  Sweet and Sour, 194, 252
  Teriyaki, 172
  White Wine, 217
Savory Brussels Sprouts, 182
Scalloped Potatoes, 247
Scrambled Eggs, 166
seafood recipes.
    See crab recipes; fish recipes;
    shrimp recipes
Sears, Barry, 56-57
sea vegetables, 108, 285

selenium, 52
self-hypnosis, 40-41, 102, 272
Sesame Bread Sticks, 256
sesame oil, 80, 109
sesame seeds, roasting, 240
shellfish recipes.
    See crab recipes; shrimp recipes
Sherried Sweet Potatoes, 249
Shiitake Gravy, 218
Shiitake Mushroom Sauce, 250
shrimp recipes
  Shrimp Bisque, 133
  Shrimp-Cashew Szechuan Stir Fry, 177
  Shrimp Creole, 173
  Shrimp Louis Salad, 144
skin
  cleansing, 103-104
  irritation, 21, 28, 48
snake venom, 35
soft drinks, 75
Sorbet, Pineapple-Ginger, 262
Souffle, Broccoli-Tofu, 151
soup recipes
  Broccoli-Soy Cheese, 129
  Cool Avocado, 202
  Cream of Asparagus, 134
  Cream of Mushroom, 136
  Cream of Tomato, 130
  Gazpacho, 130, 200
  Golden Bisque, 230
  Manhattan Fish Chowder, 135
  Puréed Carrot, 203
  Shrimp Bisque, 133
  Vegetable, 132, 201, 202
  Zucchini Bisque, 131
Southwest Lentil Salad, 235
Southwest Slaw, 207
soy cheese recipes
  Basic Omelet For Two, 163
  Broccoli Casserole, 189
  Broccoli-Soy Cheese Soup, 129
  Broccoli-Tofu Souffle, 151
  Crab and Mushroom Bake, 174
  Creamy Veggie Bake, 156
  Fish Fromage, 169
  Grilled Vegetable Salad, 142

Soy Cheese Sauce, 193
Spanish Omelet Sauce, 164
Stuffed Zucchini, 190
Tofu-Cauliflower Casserole, 160
Vegetable Omelet, 165
Zucchini Pancake, 167
soy milk, 80
Spanish Omelet Sauce, 164
Spanish Rice Salad, 238
Spiced Mixed Fries, 249
Spinach Quiche Sans Crust, 150
Spinach Salad with Dijon Dressing, 140
spirulina, 49
Split Pea Soup, 229
squash recipes.
    See also zucchini recipes
Acorn Squash Purée, 245
Butternut Squash-Orange Purée, 242
Golden Bisque, 230
Roasted Vegetables, 213
Stuffed Squash, 248
Sweet Fall Squash Medley, 244
staphylococcus, 48
Starch-Alkaline foods.
    See Alkaline-Starch foods
Steamed Cabbage, 215
stevia, 44-45, 109
Stir-Fried Kale with Garlic, 210
Stir-Fry Sauce, 251
Strawberry Cream Pie, 264
Strawberry Sauce, 269
Stuffed Squash, 248
Stuffed Zucchini, 190
subliminal tapes, 39-41
sugar
  avoidance of, 95
  starch intake and, 56, 58
  substitutes, 44-45, 79, 109, 116
Sun Chlorella, 49, 52
Super Papaya Enzyme Plus, 49
supplements, 51-53, 280
Sweet and Sour Sauce, 194, 252
sweeteners, 44-45, 79, 109, 116.
    See also sugar
Sweet Fall Squash Medley, 244

sweet potato recipes
Sherried Sweet Potatoes, 249
Spiced Mixed Fries, 249
Sweet Potato-Black-eyed
  Pea Salad, 234
Systemic Formulas, 36
Szechuan Tofu and Stir-Fried
  Vegetables, 161

Taco Salad, 237
tahini, 109
Tai Chi, 103
Tai-ra-chi, 36
tamari, 109
tea substitutes, 79
Teccino Chocolate Mint, 198
tekka, 109, 217, 250
temporomandibular joint
  (TMJ) problems, 10-11
Teriyaki Sauce, 172
Texas Caviar, 236
Therapeutic Touch, 276
Thondup, Tulku, 40
Tips, Jack, 35
TMJ (temporomandibular joint), 10-11
tobacco, 62
tofu, 109
tofu recipes
  Asparagus Quiche Sans Crust, 149
  Basic Omelet For Two, 163
  Blackened Tofu, 152
  Broccoli-Tofu Souffle, 151
  Butterscotch Mousse with
    Toasted Almonds, 196
  Cream of Asparagus Soup, 134
  Creamy Veggie Bake, 156
  Curried Tofu, 157
  Deviled Eggs, 166
  Egg Replacer Silken Omelet, 162
  Garlic-Ripe Olive Dip, 124
  Grilled Tofu Steaks, 158
  Guacamole-Tofu Dip, 128
  Indonesian Tofu, 153
  Lemon Mousse, 197
  Lemon Sauce, 193
  Lemon-Tofu Nuggets, 154

Index

Mocha Mousse with
 Toasted Pecans, 198
Oriental Broccoli Quiche Sans
 Crust, 148
Scrambled Eggs, 166
Spinach Quiche Sans Crust, 150
Szechuan Tofu and Stir-Fried
 Vegetables, 161
Tofu-Cauliflower Casserole, 160
Tofu Loaf, 158-159
Tofu-Mushroom Pancake, 155
Tofu-Onion Dip, 127
Tofu Squares, 152
Vegetable Omelet, 165
toothpaste, 110
toxins, 62
tuna, 53
tuna recipes. *See also* fish recipes
 Canned-Tuna Bake, 181
 Grilled Tuna with Teriyaki Sauce, 172
 Tuna Casserole, 178
 Tuna Salad in Stuffed Tomato, 143

umeboshi plums, 70, 109, 206

Vanilla Pudding, 263
Vegetable Omelet, 165
vegetables, classification of, 116
Vegetable Salad with
 Creamy Ranch Dressing, 141
vegetable soups, 132, 201-202, 228
vinegar, 50, 107-109
viral infections, 31-32, 50
vitamin B, 52
vitamin C, 50, 52
vitamin E, 52
Vogue Vege Base, 110

walking impairment, 5, 10
Warm Artichoke Dip, 125
water intake, 103
watermelon, 70
web sites, 277-279
weight loss, 83
Weil, Dr. Andrew, 280
wheat grass juice, 49

Whitaker, Dr. Julian, 279
White Bean-Horseradish Salad, 239
White Bean Paté, 222
White Wine Sauce, 217
Whole Wheat Biscuits, 257
Williams, David, 279
wine, effects of, 5, 8

yarrow, 49
yeast infections, systematic, 28, 35-36
The Yeast Syndrome, 28

zinc, 50
The Zone (Sears), 56-57
zucchini recipes. *See also* squash recipes
 Carrots, Zucchini and Peas, 215
 Creamy Veggie Bake, 156
 Mushroom-Zucchini Puff, 184
 Roasted Vegetables, 213
 Shrimp Creole, 173
 Stuffed Zucchini, 190
 Zucchini Bisque, 131
 Zucchini Pancake, 167
 Zucchini with Fresh Basil, 185
 Zucchini with Ginger and Cashews, 183

Order Form

QTY.	Title	Price	Can. Price	Total
	Curing The Incurable **Jacque C. Rigg**	**$18.95**	**$24.95 CN**	
	Shipping and Handling Add $3.50 for orders in the US/Add $7.50 for Global Priority			
	Sales tax (WA state residents only, add 8.6%)			
	Total enclosed			

Telephone Orders:
Call 1-800-461-1931
Have your VISA or
MasterCard ready.

INTL. Telephone Orders:
Toll free 1-877-250-5500
Have your credit card ready.

Fax Orders:
425-672-8597
Fill out this order form and fax.

Postal Orders:
Hara Publishing
P.O. Box 19732
Seattle, WA 98109

E-mail Orders:
harapub@foxinternet.net

Method of Payment:

☐   Check or Money Order

☐   VISA

☐   MasterCard

Expiration Date: _____

Card #: _____

Signature: _____

Name _____
Address _____
City _____ State _____ Zip _____
Daytime Phone (___) _____ _____

Quantity discounts are available.
Call (425) 776-3390 for more information.
Thank you for your order!